CW01429177

This book is the product of two arts and health projects run by Jackie Gay at the West Midlands Rehabilitation Centre, in collaboration with photographer Clifford Morris.

Jackie Gay is a novelist, short story writer and editor. Her second novel *Wist* was published by Tindal Street Press in July 2003.

Clifford Morris is a Fellow of the Royal Photographic Society

All proceeds from sales of this booklet will go into Trust Funds of the Rehabilitation Directorate, and they will be used to benefit staff and patients by buying goods or services which are not funded by mainstream NHS resources.

First published in 2003 by Rehab Publishing
8 Towyn Road, B13 9NA

Introduction © Jackie Gay, 2003

Copy Editor: Emma Hargrave
Typesetting: Jackie Gay

ISBN 0 9545581 0 3

Printed by
Millington York Ltd
Leighswood Road
Aldridge
Walsall
West Midlands
WS9 8AL

'*Seeing the Blue Sky*' - Stories from West Midlands Rehabilitation Centre

Edited by Jackie Gay

Contents: *Page*

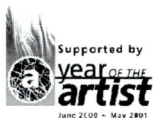

Supported by
year OF THE
artist
June 2C00 – May 2001

South Birmingham
Primary Care Trust
NHS

The editor would like to thank the Arts Council, West Midlands, and West Midlands Rehabilitation Centre for financial support of these projects. Also Clifford Morris for his wonderful pictures and Emma Hargrave for editorial and production advice. Judith Davis, Elaine Burt, Sue Roberts and Cynthia Bower from South Birmingham Primary Care Trust have all supported my work in rehabilitation and I thank them for trusting me with the opportunity.

Most of all I would like to thank the patients who have allowed me into their lives and given me their inspirational stories.

Introduction

What words strike terror into your heart? I bet the following count among them: brain damage, congenital defects, cerebral infection, spinal damage, amputation, stroke, head injury. But these things happen to ordinary people every day and it is the job of rehabilitation centres to enable people who have suffered such enormous disruptions in their lives to return to the community. The stories in this booklet came out of two writer-in-residence projects which I undertook at the West Midlands Regional Rehabilitation Centre and Moseley Hall Hospital Neuro-Rehabilitation Unit between 2001-3. A key aspect of the projects was to focus on the person as a whole, to de-medicalise them and recognise that people with disabilities also have homes, jobs, families, interests and opinions – especially about their own treatment and how best to manage their lives after the event.

Rehabilitation is defined in the dictionary as: '[to] restore [someone] to health or normal life by training and therapy after imprisonment, addiction or illness,' from the Latin 'restore to former privileges'. Before I lost my left leg above the knee in 1994 in a traumatic accident – not through imprisonment or addiction, I hasten to add – I didn't think that being able-bodied was a 'privilege', although I certainly do now. And as for restoring the privilege, that's very unlikely, no matter now much 'training and therapy' I might get. So the name of the game is adjustment; adaptation to new circumstances which can often be slow, painful and demoralising. During my own rehabilitation I became aware that the most helpful interventions often came from peers, people who have been through similar experiences and that there was a real benefit to sharing stories.

All my interviewees have had to think hard about their disabilities and their lives. It was fascinating to see how articulate people were about their own experiences and how their own phraseology illuminates their inner lives – so much more powerful than any interpretations I might make. While typing up the interviews I often found myself going back to the tape and listening carefully to record the exact phrase used and stop myself 'filling in' with the sense of the story. People found the process of both talking and writing about their situations, exchanging and reading other peoples' stories, 'inspiring' and 'excellent'. There was a real sense that patients could and did encourage each other in their rehabilitation. I hope that readers of these stories will be similarly inspired by the courage, tenacity, humour and fortitude of my interviewees and their families. For disabled people to be truly accepted for who they are and properly integrated into society then the able-bodied need to challenge their fears. For centuries disability has been associated with the loss of an essential part of a person's humanity; these stories challenge that assumption. They are the real stories of real people.

Jackie Gay
August 2003

Stuart Penn was born in Birmingham in 1978 without a left arm, right leg or left fibia. His greatest love is martial arts, which he teaches professionally. At the time of this interview he was working in a bank and hoping to be able to teach Tae Kwon Do full time – he has now achieved this aim.

I was born without a left arm, just below the elbow, so luckily I have got a bit of movement. I've got a tiny little bit of right knee, and I've got the fibia missing from my left leg which gives me the deformed foot. They're not sure why it happened, it just did. I was lucky, my parents insisted that I went to a normal school, and I had no problems. Because I was born like this I've always seen myself as being right and everyone else as wrong – it goes with my arrogant attitude!

I was very young when I first had prosthetics fitted, at first I just had a peg leg with no foot. Apparently I wouldn't go out without a shoe, so my parents taped one onto the limb. Then I had aluminium limbs, then metal or wooden ones with foam over the top. Just in the 20 plus years of my life I've gone from wearing big wooden tree-trunk legs about 10 inches wide – we'd have to buy men's trousers and they'd still be skin-tight on me – to the high-tech limbs I've got now. Before, the knee was just two metal bolts and an elastic band, I had a big leather belt to hold it on. I still have scars on my back from the constant wearing of the belt on my skin.

The Limb Centre is my second home – I've been coming here as long as I can remember. I dread to think of how many legs I've broken: hundreds, I should think, absolutely loads. Once we left the centre with this brand new, meant-to-be-indestructible leg. Within two hours I was back again; I'd shattered the knee, it was gone. I was about 11.

I was one of the first people to have an electric hand. I still use it for certain things, but a lot of the time I find it's difficult to move the muscles to get it going. I might just as well reach over. Some people are brilliant with them, though. Normally I just wear the cosmetic arm. I think the arms have come on less than the legs. People still use the claws and hooks – I remember them from when I was a kid.

Martial arts is my biggest love. I used to do judo as a child and in my teens went on to Tae Kwon Do, it seemed like a natural progression. I started judo at about nine and Tae Kwon Do at 12. I wasn't really a sporty person as a kid, but as I got more and more into Tae Kwon Do it sort of took over. When Andrew Sharpe became my prosthetist he started giving me more experimental legs, which meant I could start running – I couldn't run before I had these legs. I really got into Tae Kwon Do once I could do more. It became my passion. Andy has helped a lot and he still does, comes up with new ideas, his mind's always four steps ahead of what he's saying. I know these are the sturdiest legs I can get. I trust Andy when he says, 'This is the knee that'll cope best.' I've got an Otto Bock knee and a suspension system on my foot.

Next year I'm starting up my own karate class. At the moment I teach in Cambridgeshire. Birmingham is saturated with karate clubs so a group of us travel down and teach twice a week. When I teach kids, I always have a question and answer session where they can ask me about my limbs. They have to learn a bit of Korean for Tae Kwon Do, so I let them ask five questions about me, but then they've got to answer five questions in Korean. I just say that I'm normal and that they've got too many arms and legs as far as I'm concerned. That seems to go down well. I've done a few competitions and got a couple of silvers in mainstream, able-bodied Tae Kwon Do. I'd like to take it further, see if I can get a European or world title. I've become a bit of an urban legend, this guy with an arm and leg missing. When I teach around the country there's always people whispering, 'I heard there's someone with a leg missing . . .'

I go by the same rules as everyone else, I don't get any preferential treatment. I'm a second dan black belt*. Internationally you're a master at fourth dan, in England it's sixth dan – we make it harder and do it properly! When I first passed my black belt I was there with about 200 people and I was in the top 13. I was marked exactly the same as everyone else, which showed that I was quite good at it as well.

I do a lot of running, sprinting and cycling. I play squash as well, and tennis, hill running. In Tae Kwon Do you do a lot of circuit training – fitness is a lot to do with martial arts. Before I could run I used to go into the corner when the others were doing circuit training and my instructor would get me doing sit-ups and press-ups. Then I got an earlier version of this leg and realised I could run on it, but my fitness wasn't there for running. So I started dashing around in a circle until my fitness went or my leg got sore. It really helped when the Silopos socks came in. They're gel socks instead of cotton ones. I can't remember how on earth I used to get on with just cotton socks.

My parents and my instructor have been the most influential people in my life. I used to see my instructor do things and I'd think, 'I can do that.' No one has ever tried to hold me back. Andy always wants to help. If I told him I was going to become a bungee jumper and I wanted a leg to stay on he'd do one for me. At Oak Tree Lane Centre you can say, 'I want to do this,' and they won't try and talk you out of it.

Editor's note:
Stuart is pictured on the front cover of this booklet
*He is now a third dan black belt

In 2000 Michael Perks had an infection on his spine and was paralysed from the waist down. He spent seven months in the QE and then four months in rehab at Moseley Hall.

At the QE they were very, very pessimistic about me walking again. They thought I might end up tetraplegic; the surgeon said, 'We've got to see whether we can save your trunk.' What can you do? He was pessimistic and I was optimistic. I spent seven months in bed, 24 hours a day. All I could see were the tops of the trees. When they first gave me a wheelchair I was down the corridor and out into the open air not realising that all I'd got on was my underpants . . . and it was October! Fresh air was fantastic. But I always said to them, 'If I see so much as a flicker in my toe then you'd better get out of my way.' I couldn't feel anything in my legs but used to get spasms and I thought, 'Well, something's working, something's coming back in.'

Early on, my wife thought she was going to lose me. I was down, depressed, weak, on so many drugs; like a shrivelled old man. They ran out of veins in my arms and had to put a Hickman line in my chest. But then, when I was at probably my lowest point, Amie, my son's partner's daughter came to see me with Adrian, my son. She brought me a photograph of herself in a green frame. I put it at the bottom of my bed and made a pledge that I'd make myself better. She was only seven at the time; she couldn't do anything, didn't know what to say, but she was there. We're mates now – she hasn't got a grandad, only me; she's the light of my life she is.

When I got to Moseley, within 12 weeks I went from being in bed, to a wheelchair, to the Zimmer frame, to elbow crutches to walking. I was wheeled in and walked out - they called me the Miracle Man. Ian, my physio, was brilliant, brilliant. The first day I had a shower, I cried – fantastic. Now I've got a Hartshill rectangle in my spine holding it together; some days I'm in a lot of pain but on others I forget it's there. What do they say – laugh in the face of adversity?

Recovery, rehabilitation: it's mental as well as physical. In Moseley, there's a camaraderie. When you're in rehab you've got to encourage people. You'd see a guy walking with sticks and you'd say, 'Hang on, yesterday you only walked to there . . .' and he'd say, 'Did I?' We'd purposely notice, you see. We knew each other well, what people liked to eat and we'd tell the staff, 'Excuse me, this guy doesn't like this, and he won't eat it.' These were people who couldn't say it for themselves. It's comradeship really.

When I first got my wheelchair I'd come out of Ward 3 and turn into that long corridor and pull myself along with my feet. It took me 35 minutes the first time. Every day I did it faster, the power was coming back into my legs. When I could take a few steps I said to Ian, 'We've got to keep mum about this,' because I wanted to surprise my wife. Then I said to Adrian, 'This Sunday, bring Mom up on Sunday night.' He said, 'What for?' and I said, 'It would be nice for you to all come together.' When they arrived I went to the toilet in my wheelchair, got my Zimmer out then, and I walked back in, you see. That was the first time I'd walked for nine months.

From my room on Ward 3 to the gymnasium on Hillcrest it was 936 paces. I'd do that at least three times a day. Jez – one of the physios – he used to call me the Walking Man. I've got a certificate from the staff and patients saying, 'You've earned the right to escape from Hillcrest.' I knew I was on my way – a new life. People don't realise what's been taken away from you. Now I'm walking on my own two feet, I'm independent again, playing golf even.

Mentally you think, 'How am I going to cope?' But I don't need much motivation. Fortitude is important – thankfully that was part of my personality. I never ever gave up the fact that I was going to walk again. I *was* going to walk again. The doctors should use me as an example and say, 'We were pessimistic that Michael would ever walk again but now he's running, virtually.'

You're plunged into a society that a lot of people consider to be that of outcasts. I think it's a sad shame, those attitudes. I go the other way: if I see someone in a wheelchair I'll go over and talk to them. I've become more outspoken since my illness: if something's wrong I'll say so. But others have been very, very kind and caring – if I go to the club people will go out of their way to get a seat with arms for me because they know I like a seat with arms.

People said to me, 'What's the first thing you're going to do when you go home?' I said, 'Walk with bare feet on wet grass.' Now I hardly ever wear shoes in the house, I like to feel the carpet under my feet, go out into the garden. No matter how tough the going gets, you must never give up and never be afraid to ask for help when you need it. The reason you're in rehab is because you need help. I still walk barefoot on wet grass – it's beautiful and I couldn't have done it without a great deal of help and TLC.

Michelle Green was born in Birmingham in 1973. In January 1996 she was run over by a hit-and-run driver, damaging her hips, pelvis and left leg. She eventually decided to have the leg amputated in September 1999 and is now learning to walk again.

My childhood was all right, but my mum and dad divorcing did affect me – I was a really quiet child, completely different to what I am now. I was happy to grow up, wouldn't want to go back there. I'm gay; I was 18 when I came out. All these girls were rushing around after boys and I just wasn't bothered. It used to get on top of me because I thought I didn't want to be gay, but then I nearly got killed and now if anyone has a problem it's their problem.

When the accident happened I was living with a friend, Clint, in Newtown. A couple of nights before I dreamed that I'd drowned and I was watching my family at my funeral. That particular day, I didn't want to go out. My mom phoned me up that morning – she never phoned me early in the day – and said, 'Are you all right?' and I said, 'Yes, why?' and she didn't say anything. She'd dreamed that I'd died and somebody had given her a baby in replacement. I was supposed to be going out that night but I was being sick all day, there was just something . . . I couldn't find any clean socks, only one green sock and one orange sock, and I said to Clint, 'If I have an accident you'd better take them off me.' Then ten minutes later I was run over.

We were waiting for a bus outside the Barton Arms. We'd been waiting a while and then saw a bus going the other way and Clint said, 'Let's go and catch that instead.' All I remember is him going to cross the road and hearing three massive bangs, going right through me, and then silence. I knew something bad had happened. To me, the ambulance was there within seconds. I was swearing and screaming with an

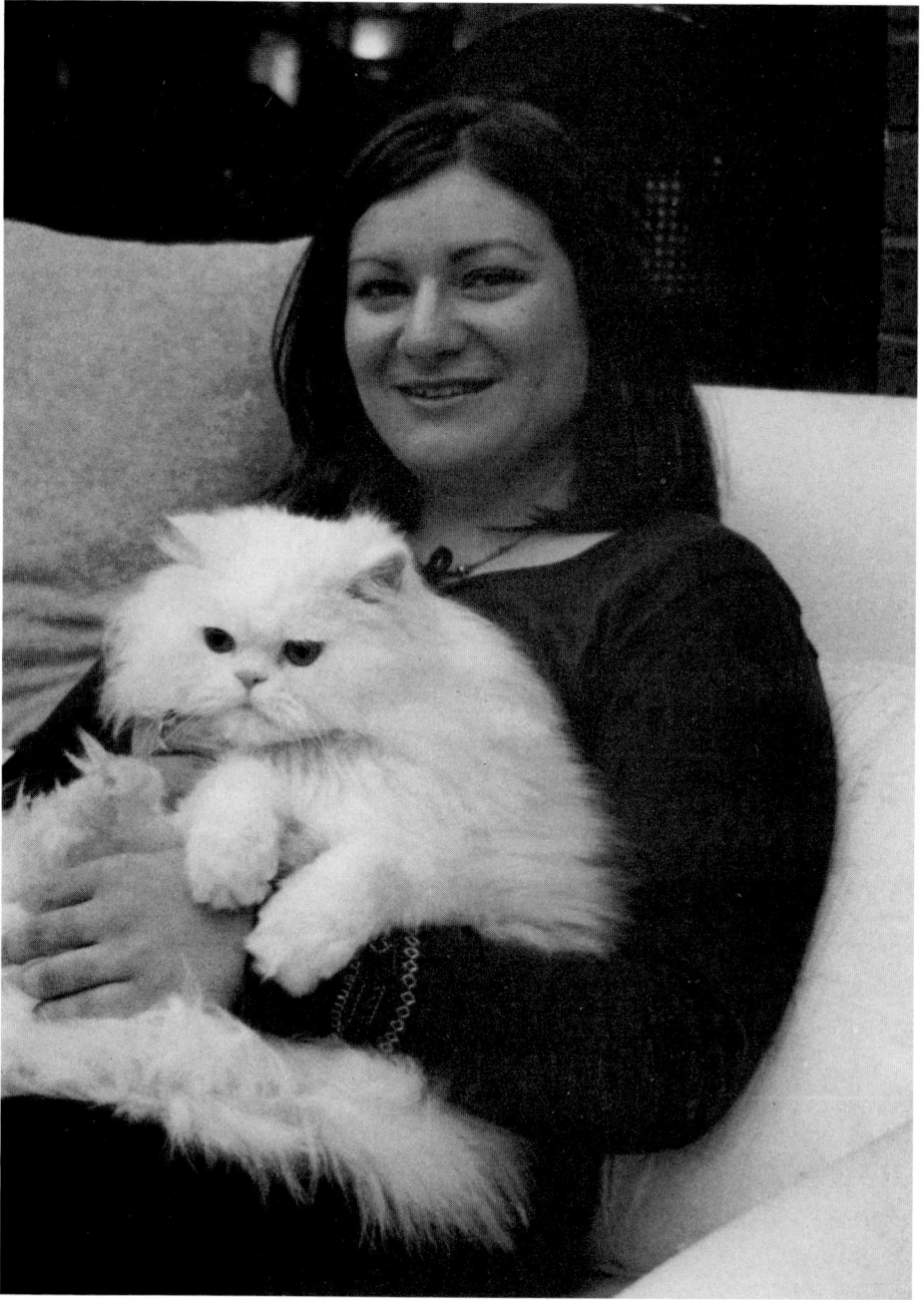

unbelievable pain in my back. The leg was torn at the thigh, the main artery ripped and they severed an artery in theatre as well. But my pelvis was the main problem: the 'wing' was sticking right out and both the hips were broken. I went straight into theatre and was in there for 14 hours; I was really, really ill. I had 78 units of blood that first night, it was just going in and coming straight out of the wound. I was having a lot of drugs and hallucinating, but it got to the stage where I was really and truly bad. It turned out I had a ruptured gall bladder and septicaemia.

They were really negative from day one about the outlook over my leg. I felt like they'd written me off. At that point I couldn't even lift my head up, I was like a rag doll. It annoys me when I see these programmes about people in intensive care and they're drugged up, look really at peace and they wake up and suddenly they're better. I mean, you've got to learn to walk, talk again, never mind anything else. I remember learning to swallow: the ward sister gave me some water and couldn't find the hole where the drink goes, I was panicking, saying, 'What do I do?' I remember jelly being like rock, trying to swallow it for the first time.

When they discharged me I still had my leg, but I couldn't put weight on it. I'd get in the bath and it would turn upside down. My girlfriend said, 'If you want my opinion I think you should have your leg amputated,' and I remember getting so mad, if anybody even mentioned it. But the blood supply was really bad – a blister on my toe took three or four months to heal, I had to be careful everywhere. I really missed just being able to throw myself on the bed or the sofa and not worry about hurting myself. People said, 'I don't know why you're so against it,' but it was just the thought of it. You're brought up with it, in society. I was worried about waking up after the op thinking, 'What have I

15

done?' But I'd tried absolutely everything, had about 15 operations. I was so tired, so exhausted, it could only be better.

I came into the limb fitting centre and the doctor said that because my hips were so badly damaged he wasn't sure if I'd be able to walk on a leg, but he said, 'We'll try our best.' It's brilliant now, best decision I ever made and I don't regret it at all. I did underestimate the physio, because I hadn't walked for three years. They said, 'It's going to be hard work getting up walking again.' It was such a shock to the system. They couldn't get me into the PPAM-aid because I had oedema, there was blood coming through my bandage and it felt terrible, barbaric. That first week was just awful, but after that I was raring to go, do anything they suggested.

Even now, if I get ill with a virus or a temperature I turn into a quivering wreck. All I can think of is intensive care, it just brings everything back. It scares you to death, being that ill. You feel like a nutter. When you tell people they don't really get it. But when you know what the pain is like, the mental thing, collars round your neck, tubes, metal work, not even being able to move your head, you think, 'How did I do that?'

I seem to spend my whole life getting over things – I thought that coming out as gay was the big thing in my life and then I had the accident and lost my leg and now I think, 'What's next?' Nothing surprises me now. I think I've gone more selfish since the accident – not selfish, but I used to be one of these people you could walk all over, but now if someone upsets me I just say. Before I used to do what other people wanted, do things to please other people. Having an accident like that puts things into perspective.

Rod Palmer was born in Hampshire in 1944 and moved to Birmingham when he was two. He worked as an estimating engineer until he was made redundant in 1999. Both his legs have been amputated below the knee.

My dad came out of the navy and we moved up to Birmingham – I'm bred but not born in Brum. I was diagnosed diabetic at age two and have used insulin all my life. I don't know any other way of life. It never stopped me from playing sports at school, or getting a job after I left – I wouldn't let it.

I lost the left leg in 1987. One day I got in the shower and there was blood between my toes. The next morning an infection had run from the toe to the knee. It happened very quickly. Being a diabetic I knew that this would be serious. I said to the doctor, 'Doc, you'd better have a look at my foot, because it's in a bad way.' It was just black and he said, 'I'm going to take you in straight away – you do realise that you'll lose your leg?' I said, 'I know that.'

Not once did I ever ask, 'Why me?' But I had a peculiar experience in hospital. A cousin of mine is a born-again Christian, and he came to see me the day before they were going to amputate. He said, 'We've come to pray for you,' and I thought, 'I'm not into this,' but he was very serious about it. He started to pray. I was lying on my side and saw the most brilliant white light – up my body, over my shoulders, my head. And then I wasn't even in the hospital, but in this meadowland with hundreds of people all walking across dressed in clothes of biblical times. And in front of me were three men, walking by this stream. As I was catching up with them they turned. The man in the middle was Jesus. Then I was back in my room, in bed in the hospital. Mom and Dad came to see me that same afternoon and Dad said to

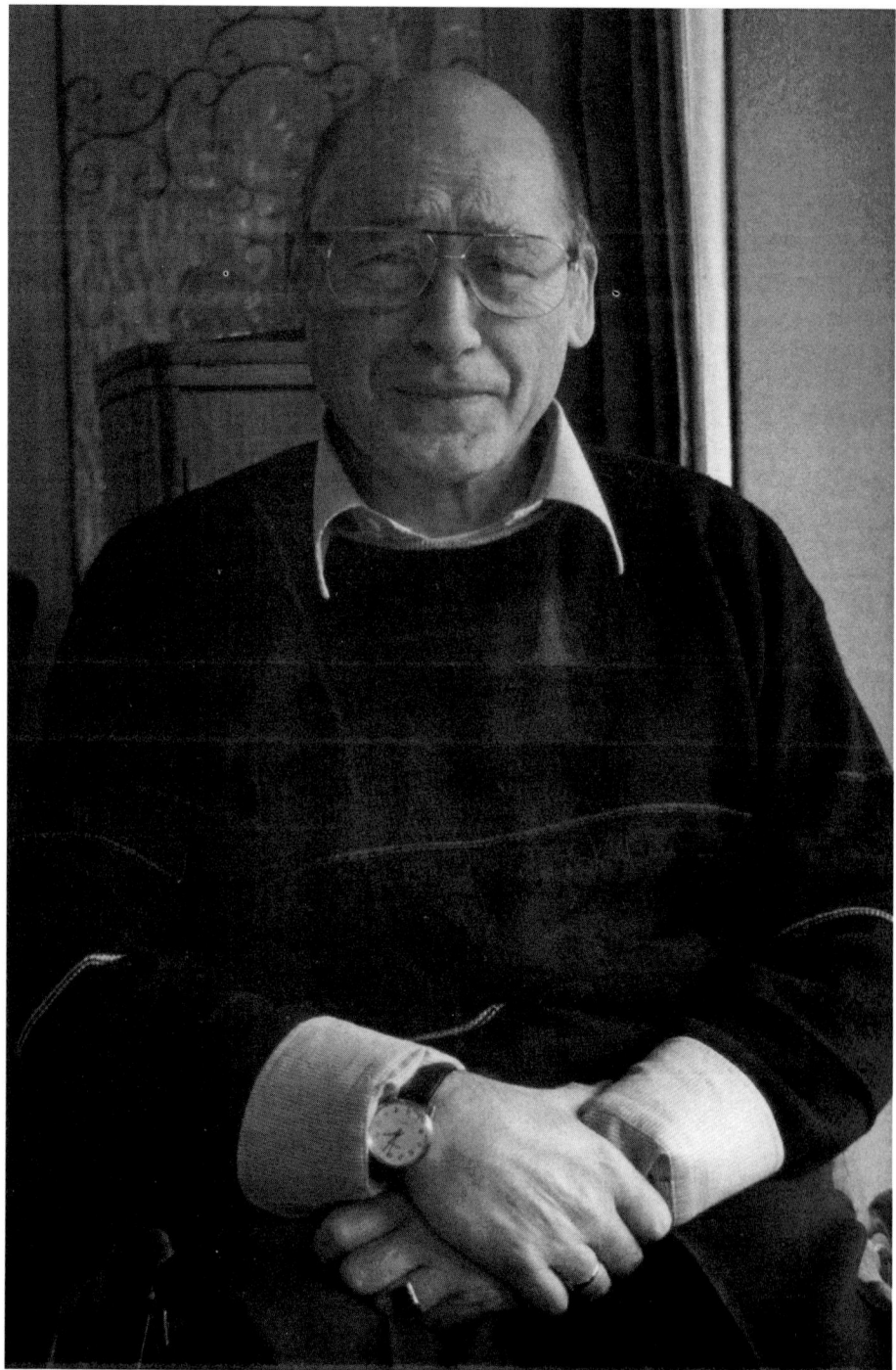

the ward sister, 'What drugs have you given to my son?' She said, 'What made you ask that?' He said, 'Because his attitude has completely changed, he's not worrying about losing his leg.' She said, 'We haven't given him anything because he's refused, but we've noticed the change too.' What I'd got after that experience was peace of mind, absolute peace of mind.

I still get quite emotional thinking about it. My doctor at the time came to see me and I remember him saying, 'Have you accepted your amputation?' I said yes and he said, 'That's good, because once your mind's accepted it the rest of the body will follow, and ti it's the best way.'

I went back to work on one good leg and a pair of crutches, before I even got my prosthesis. They were glad to see me back. Then three years later the big toe on my other leg went off colour. I was admitted into Selly Oak to have a vascular operation. On the Saturday the consultant came round and I said, 'What are the chances of success?' He looked at me as if he didn't want to answer. So I said, 'I know there won't be 100 per cent, so what about 70?' He said, 'No.' I said, '50 per cent?' 'No.' I said, 'You can give me a 25 per cent chance of success?' He said, 'No.' I said, 'Right, take it off, get rid of it.' I've met guys at the limb centre who'd had three, four, five of these vascular operations and still had their leg amputated, the trouble being they amputated above the knee. I thought, 'No; no way.'

My prosthetist was Fred Rose. I was with him from 1987 until he retired. I'll always remember him saying to me, 'We can't replace what you've lost, but with my knowledge and your endeavours we'll get you back on your feet.' Great guy. I remember once in physio they had a set of steps, and the physios were telling us amputees, 'You get your crutches, and you go up onto the first step and you bring your crutches up.' But us guys were having all sorts of problems, so in the end we all ganged together and said, 'What we want is one of you physios to immobilise one of your legs and try it yourselves.' They got some old bandage and tied this girl's leg back and gave her the crutches. She couldn't do it, wasn't half in a mess. She said, 'I've suddenly realised how difficult it is,' and she appreciated what we were going through.

I got clamped in my wheelchair on a ferry once, coming back from the Isle of Wight. The ferry was really crowded and my mates said, 'Are you going to come and sit with us or will you stop in your wheelchair?' I said, 'I'll stop in my wheelchair, I'm quite comfortable.' A crew member came over to me and said I'd have to be clamped to the deck for safety reasons. I said, 'OK, fair enough.' We got back to Portsmouth harbour and I'm sitting in my wheelchair watching everybody get off and then I realised that the gangplank was coming back on board. From the quay I heard one of my friends shout, 'Stop that ferry, our mate in a wheelchair's still on board.' Next thing I know the gangplank has swung back round, two crew members and two of my mates come running across the deck. I was seconds away from going back to the Isle of Wight.

There's no alternative to being level-headed about what's happened. If you don't accept it what are you going to do? Destroy the world or something? When a surgeon says to you, 'Look, if you keep your leg, you die; if we take the leg away, you live,' there's no choice. There are many physical limitations to what I can do, and everything isn't fine. But my family have been very good to me. You've got to cope. This isn't a practice run – it's all you've got, you've got to make the most of it.

In April 2001 Jan Mieczynski was struck down by Guillain-Barré syndrome (GBS), an acute disease of the nervous system. He came to Moseley Hall in December 2001. Jan married his long-term partner Beverley in the chapel at the hospital; they have two daughters, Fay (12) and Heather (seven).

Beverley: Jan came home after a fry-up and felt a bit sick, but he was OK the day after. Towards the end of the week he said he felt like he had the flu. The next day we went to A&E and they said it was probably a muscular spasm, then possibly kidney stones. But he got worse again, and we called an ambulance. I told the hospital that something else was happening and they said it was a panic attack. We waited from four in the afternoon until 12 at night to see a doctor and by the time he came Jan's lips were blue. He was deteriorating as we were watching him – my Jan was lying on this bed and being slowly taken away from me. We were sent to the QE for tests. The next day Jan couldn't even speak. All of a sudden he just stopped breathing on me and was given a lumber puncture – I really thought he'd died at that minute – and then they moved him up to intensive care. The doctor said to me, 'You're looking at 48 hours – if you're lucky – the way he's going now, if he has got GBS.' Jan was totally paralysed, only his eyes were moving, and his head, slowly. They sent him for a MRI and he went into a coma for two weeks.

Jan: I can't remember any of this. The last thing that's clear to me is going to the Lickeys on the Saturday before. One in 40,000 people get GBS and I'm the worst case the QE have ever seen. All I can remember of those days is the most horrendous hallucinations. They felt like they were so real. In one of them I knew I was in hospital, but they'd

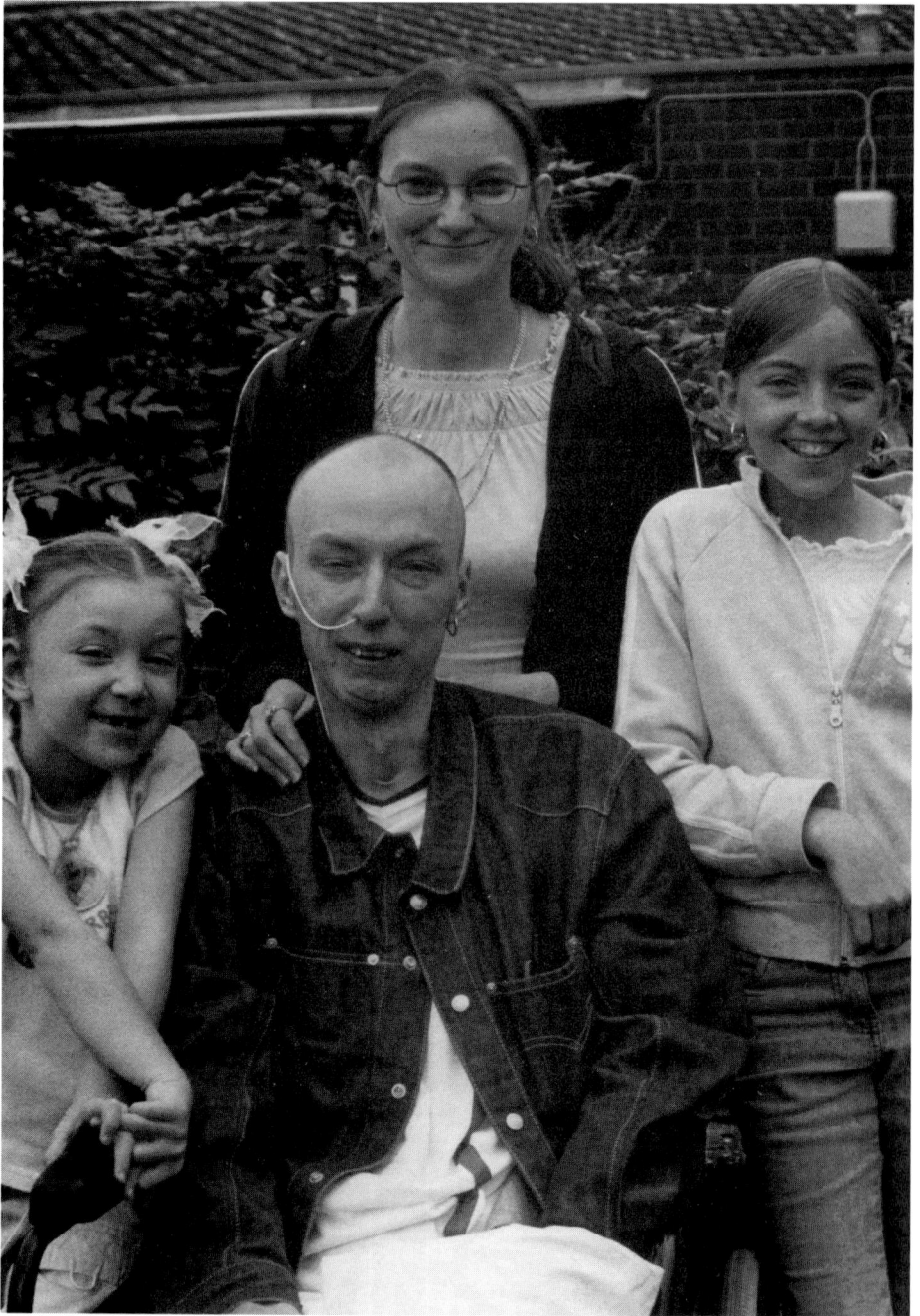

put me in a caravan and a couple of burglars came in. I was paralysed; one of them was putting glue in my eyes.

Beverley: At the time, Jan was having gel put in his eyes. He couldn't shut them for two weeks, so you can imagine the dryness. His pupils stopped dilating – that's how paralysed he was. The staff told us that if he did come round, then he might not even know who he is. I was just gutted, I couldn't believe it. Heather was only four. I could see Jan's body shutting down before my eyes, and slowly I saw it coming back. Then one day he nodded when a nurse said, 'Jan, can you hear me?' – I fell to pieces; thought, 'Thank God.' They gave Jan some plasma and he started to come round; he was in critical care from May to September.

Jan: Dr Asar had seen me when I was in intensive care. He told me that he'd thought, 'This lad's in trouble ...' I had all my faculties when I came round, but I could only blink. I didn't speak for months.

Beverley: His face would light up when I went in, all the machines would go mad. The nurses said, 'He knows you're here.' When he was in a coma I took the girls in, just told them their dad was asleep. They'd cried when they saw him going into the ambulance, so if Jan was going to die I didn't want that to be their last memory. The nurse was brilliant: she hid all the wires so all the girls could see was their dad. They cried, both ran out crying, but they came back in after five minutes and they came round and he was just their dad. One day the nurse was really excited; she said, 'I've been crying all morning.' He'd moved his hands. Everyone was so emotional. Then he started getting his strength back, doing the exercises. Another high was when I felt his diaphragm move for the first time: he was breathing again. He couldn't manage it for long, but I thought, 'Yes, it's coming back.' We were chuffed when he started waving, said to the girls, 'Look, Dad's waving goodbye.'

Jan: The speech therapist came and gave me a speaking valve to attach to my tracheotomy. We had a laugh with that: it kept shooting off across the bed. I made Bev cry. The speech therapist said, 'Just say a couple of easy words; one, two, three,' but instead of saying that I said, 'I love you, Beverley.' The speech therapist – her eyes just glazed up straight away. It was a shock for everyone. I said to Bev's dad, 'Thanks for coming, Roy,' and he looked at me and filled up – although he says he didn't! But it took so long.

Beverley: It was such an achievement. The girls hadn't spoken with their dad for six months. Fay knew what was going on, that he was very poorly. Whereas Heather, when he was in critical care, was saying, 'When does my dad have his tea?' But Fay knew. They were golden.

Jan: Not long after I got to Moseley, around Christmas time, I ended up getting septicaemia again. Helen, my OT, got me home for Christmas day – I ended up making her my godmother because of that! And after I got over all the infections we got married here, on Valentine's Day. Reverend Lynne married us – she's a good friend now, a proper friend. During this we've lost a lot of friends. I was from a large circle, and there's one especially who never comes to see me. I saved his life a couple of months before I got ill: dragged him out the river in the dead of night when we were fishing. It has hurt me. I just want people to keep in touch.

Beverley: Jan's got a bit of feeling in his ankles now; he has progressed since he's been here. But we've just found out about a problem with his kidneys. We were distraught. There was no consoling us the day we found out, you can imagine. It's not to do with the GBS, apparently; they've never known anything like it. The doctor was gutted, telling us: you could see it in his face. There are a few options, though. I said to Jan, 'All through this you've proved them wrong, don't give up now.' Jan can move his feet a bit now. All I heard in the QE was, 'Can you wiggle your toes?' and I prayed for the day he could, because I knew that was what they were looking for. If you can move your toes you should get some mobility back. Now we've found out that parts of his brain are swollen as well, just to top it all. So we've been fighting the GBS, not knowing what the treatments are for the other conditions. But we know we're lucky. When you go back to those first few days, you realise that. We're unlucky because of what happened to us, but we're lucky in what we've gained back, and that's the only way you can look at it. It's been a learning curve, especially for the girls. They've both changed so much. Before all this, we had to drag Heather to the doctor's, screaming. Now, she wants to be a doctor, she's just there. Their school reports have been brilliant. Fay's had her SATs and I haven't helped her at all. She got her books out and got on with it. We're so proud of her. And my family have helped me so much; every one of them has done a different job. They've kept the stability there for the kids, their routine and normal life.

Jan: If it wasn't for Beverley and my dad and Roy and everyone I wouldn't have done this. They've been here every single day. The girls are so proud of me – just little things that I do. It was Heather's birthday and I bought her a card from the shop down here. My writing is a bit scribbly still, but you can just about read it. I sent her this card and she said to everyone, 'This is my bestest card because it's got my dad's writing in it.'

Beverley: I thought: 'I could just hug her to death.' Every time he comes home she gets the card down and reads it. Last week he made them a cake; they loved it. He can come out in the car and pick the girls up from school with me now. We went to Webbs the other day: our first outing on our own with the wheelchair. We got there and there's a bloody car show on! Coachloads of people. I said, 'Stuff it,' and we went in for two hours, then had a picnic in the car. We walked round Webbs smiling, chatting and laughing and we were happy doing it. We are happy. Nothing's going to hold us back now. I keep saying to Jan, 'Any chance you get to do anything in life now, you do it.'

Jan: My advice to people in rehab – and I know it sounds like a cliché – is just to be thankful for what you've got left and work on that. Build on that. But I have been through hell. I was there, knocking on the grim reaper's door, but he wasn't having it for some reason.

Beverley: He said to me, 'Why wasn't I taken?' And I said, 'Because you've still got a life, Jan.'

Jan: My family do need me.

Editor's note

Jan is now out of hospital and settled back happily at home with his family. He uses a standing frame daily to straighten his legs and strengthen his body and some feeling has returned to his feet.

Betty Munro was born in Hoylake, Cheshire, in 1926 and spent her childhood in Dorridge. She has lost both her legs due to poor circulation and rehabilitated at Moseley Hall Hospital where she became a founder member of the Hopping Mad Club.

I joined the Wrens when I left school, on D-Day in 1944, June 6th. It was lovely. I don't like being shut in. Had I been a boy I would have joined the navy. I was a signaller, a flag wagger, and then a motor transport driver, three-ton lorries. I left because I'd got a job to go to, driving for the government car service. I worked for about 16 years, here in Birmingham. We drove civil servants, tax collectors, the press, things like that. We provided transport for the Queen. Then I went to Geneva for four months with the World Health Organisation, then came back and got married. I worked at Stanford & Mann Stationers at Birmingham University, and I was there 16 years – I only went for five minutes! That was nice, being in the university – I love students, the young. I worked until I was 66.

I was always healthy except for the cancer. They don't know how things start, but I fell over and landed on this tin in my shopping bag, and when I got up I was black around my breast. It seemed to start from there. I went into the General on 15th December – my husband's birthday – had it removed on the 16th, came home Christmas Eve, showered and we went to a party. I had seven people to lunch on Christmas Day. Life went on normally, I went back to work. The surgeon was marvellous, he wanted to see me in my clothes and said, 'Which one is it?' I said, 'Oh come on, you took it off,' and he said, 'I can't tell.' The first thing that Sister said to me is, 'Oh, he's left you some cleavage.' I could still wear low dresses.

I have a right-below knee and a left-above knee amputation.

The right leg came off in 1996. I call my legs B & Q. I'd had ulcers through poor circulation, it got so I couldn't walk very well. The district nurse and everybody were wonderful, but they can't do miracles. The ulcers got worse and worse and worse, my leg was just covered in them, all over. The operation was at Selly Oak and then I went to Moseley Hall for rehabilitation. I'd worked there as a volunteer, talking to people, reading cards and letters for them, writing, feeding people who couldn't feed themselves. I had a pal for years – same age as me – who was paralysed from the neck down and I used to take her out. She's the one who makes you feel positive. She'd sit there, unable to do a thing, and one day she said, 'Aren't I lucky? If I was blind I wouldn't be able to see all this.' It was spring and there were dancing lambs and daffodils. That's a philosophy I've always kept to.

When I got to Moseley Hall I thought, 'Help is here for us, the thing is to listen to what they're telling you.' They show you what to do, how to get in and out of bed, the bath, a chair; then you won't get caught out at home. Elsie was 91 when she had her amputation, she cut me down to size. We were in the corridor and we stopped and had a chat. I was asking about her leg and she said, 'I don't know whether I'm going to have a leg.' I said, 'Oh, we're all going to have legs.' She leaned over and prodded me and said, 'I don't know how old you are but I'm 91.' I felt about two. She does have a leg, though, and walks now at 94. There was a Job's comforter in the ward; he said, 'It might go to the other leg.' I said, 'This time next year you'll be driving your car,' and he was.

We talked about setting up some kind of club after we were discharged from Moseley Hall. It was Doctor Rowe who wrote to the *Lancet* and he christened it the Hopping Mad Club. We're very lucky to be given a room and tea and so on. Other places have said, 'We'd love to start a club, but where?' They do try and put people with amputations in the ward where we meet. I go into Moseley Hall on Ring and Ride and I meet people and tell them to come to the Hopping Mad Club and ask us things, come and see what people *can* do, three or four years later. This is the big thing. Not next week or month – I don't expect you to be doing things then, but you've got to think longer term. I like to prove to people that things can be done. David went back to playing golf, he hit the ball very well.

I had time to think about my life after the amputation and I thought, 'Well, if it's going to take this pain away, then good.' Nothing can be worse than pain 24 hours a day. A lot comes down to whether you're positive. Some people want to stay in bed, but you don't have your lunch at home in bed, do you? You sit at a table with a knife and fork. If you get out of bed you feel better. My mother used to say, 'You die in bed, come on.'

On the left leg I had an ulcer on the ankle and it wouldn't heal. Initially I had a bypass, 103 stitches, but that didn't work. I've still got the scars now. I find that a bit difficult because the artificial limb rubs on those scars. I'm not moaning, but I didn't think about it at the time. Anyway, I'm waiting for a new leg now. It's difficult to get the wheelchair in the car at the moment. When I get my other leg I shall be able to stand and get in the car, and get a wheelchair at Tesco or Waitrose or wherever. At the moment I have to use the Ouija board – as I call it – to transfer. I get myself up, dressed, showered. Undressed at night. I cook, I shop. I cooked pheasant the week before last. I like nice food, we're having five for Christmas.

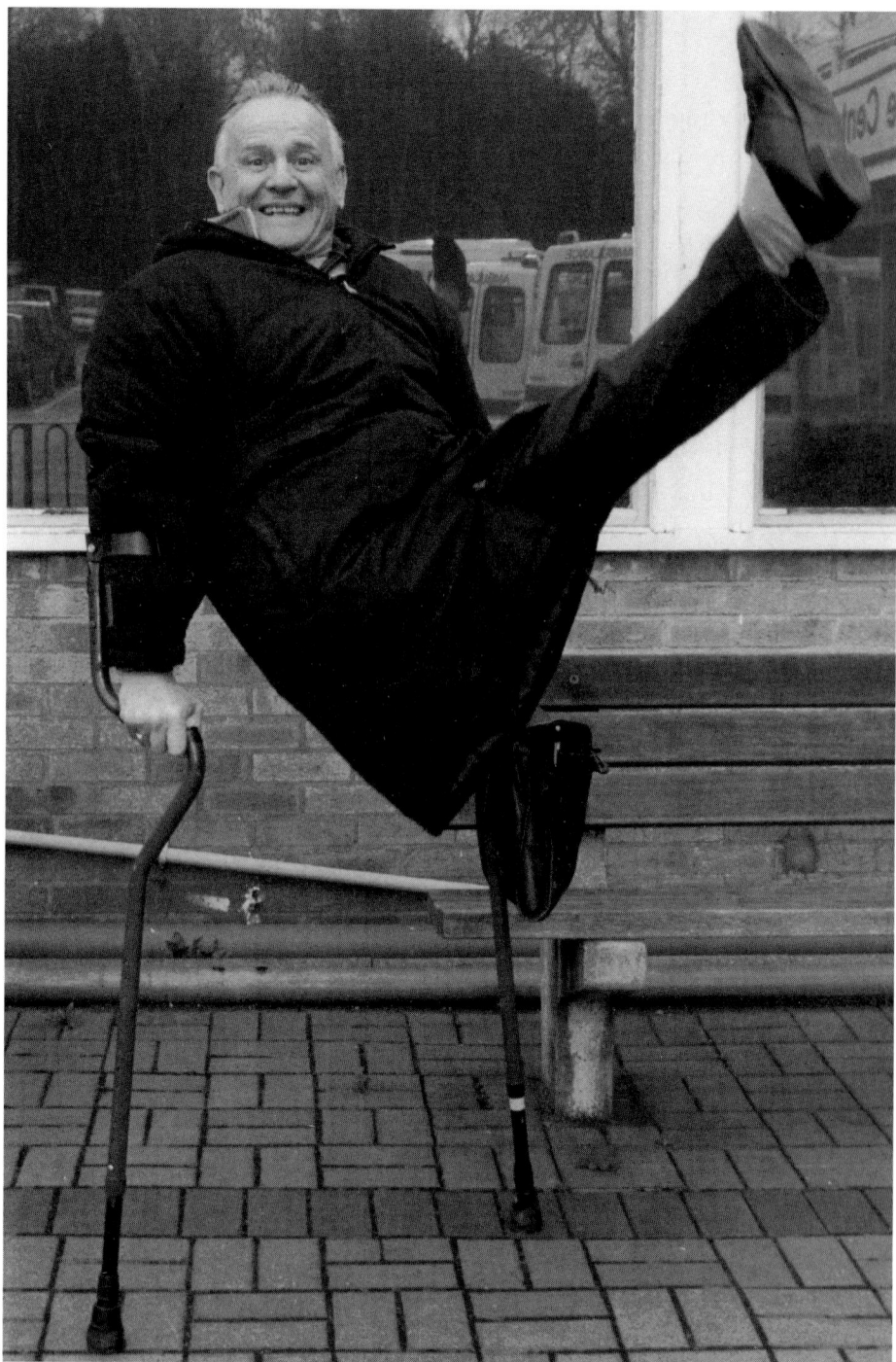

Brian Cleaver was born in 1938 in Birmingham. He became an amputee at the age of four after falling into a hollow full of broken glass. 24 hours later gas gangrene had set in – there was no penicillin available for civilians in wartime – and his right leg was amputated. Brian was the first above knee amputee to complete the London Marathon on crutches and, after a full and varied career, including working as an information officer at Birmingham Disability Information Centre, he is now happily retired.

I can't remember having two legs, but do remember the operating theatre in the General Hospital and can still to this day see those lights. For years after I lost my leg I used to dream that I could fly – aborigines would tell you there's something in that, a compensation thing – but I had a pretty normal childhood. My father taught me to use crutches using two broomsticks, I immediately went out and tried to do one of these pirouettes and finished up with a broken nose. My mom treated me with 'healthy neglect' and used to say 'stop leaving dents in the pavement' if I fell over. I wasn't cushioned. I remember one guy – Terry Hughes his name was – whipped me with privet strands and really marked me up, I had great welts across my face. Kids used to pinch my crutches and make me hop. But I got over that.

I get around easier on crutches and am always looking for non-standard ones. It's only in the last 15–18 years that I've had decent limbs, I'm on the Iceross socket now. I always knock my legs about and they become scrappers after 2 or 3 years. Even though I've stopped running now I still do a lot of walking on crutches. I'm the only man in the country to have a pair of titanium crutches, a new shape that is much more ergonomically suitable to my needs, and recently I've found some shock absorbers made in Wolverhampton, and become a test-bed for those

In 1982 I had an accident. I ran a scrap business in Wednesbury. I was piling a load of iron borings up in the yard. The only good tractor we had was started by putting a screwdriver across the battery terminals, I'd got a weight on the accelerator and the tractor jumped into gear. I was sitting on the wheel and went round with it. I can remember being crushed like a beetle, crunching like that. I broke all my ribs, perforated my lungs, broke a collarbone – didn't even dent my leg. I don't know how long I was out but I remember waking up, looking at the sky and saying 'you ent having me' to the Good Lord. I crawled to the phone and they rushed me into Dudley Guest Hospital. Recovering from that I started trotting about on my wooden crutches and I said to my wife, 'I'm going to do this run in Wolverhampton' which was five miles. It knocked hell out of me, but after the blisters healed up I went on to do a half marathon and it's gone on from there. I did 17 marathons and around 120 half marathons. It started off to get my lungs working again. During the 10 years I did marathons I think I was an inspirational runner, people thought, 'I'm not letting that one-legged bloke beat me,' and found new energy.

When I'm running, if a child has said, 'Oh look, Mom, that man's got one leg,' and the Mom's gone, 'Ssshsh', I've always stopped and said, 'Don't shush them, I have got one leg' – and the next one-legged person they see, they'll not make a comment. The only time I've felt insulted was during a run outside Stafford Prison and a woman who was directing her husband taking photographs shouted, 'Get one of *this*.' So I stopped and said, '*This* is a person, and you should be ashamed of yourself.' My shoulders are broad.

My running has been my greatest achievement. We all take out of the pot of life and some of us don't give back. I feel I've given back through my running. I've been to America four times and belong to a wonderful club wonderful club called the Achilles Track Club, which gives the opportunity to anybody to have a go at doing a marathon. Anyone – no matter what their disability. Everyone should do the New York Marathon. On the Brooklyn Bridge they have to put mats down because you can see through to the water, so you have to watch your crutches don't slip through the grids. You meet all sorts of people shouting, 'Way to go, Achilles.' In 1988 I met a lady called Zoe Koploweitz, a New Yorker, she has cerebal palsy and takes all day to do a marathon. She's very gutsy but the distinguishing thing about her is that she smiles. 'Disabled people don't smile enough,' she says. I admire her because she was told to sit in her wheelchair and fade away, and she made a decision not to do that. When she does the New York Marathon she's taken through Harlem by the Guardian Angels during the night.

I still think that disabled people aren't treated as equals. It's better now than it's ever been but disabled people are seen as 'non-citizens' who can't play a full role in society because of their disability. I always say to amputees, 'Once you get it right in your head, there's nothing you can't do.' But there's still a long way to go – there will always be prejudice. When it does occur you should stamp on it. I think that when you lose a limb people think that you've lost all your faculties. I always say to people 'you can't catch one-leg-itis' but then again it could happen to you tomorrow.

I forecast the weather with my phantom sensations. I can't say what's going to happen but if I get them really bad then the weather's going to change dramatically. When people ask me what happened to my leg I say, 'I lost it as a child – and I never found it.'

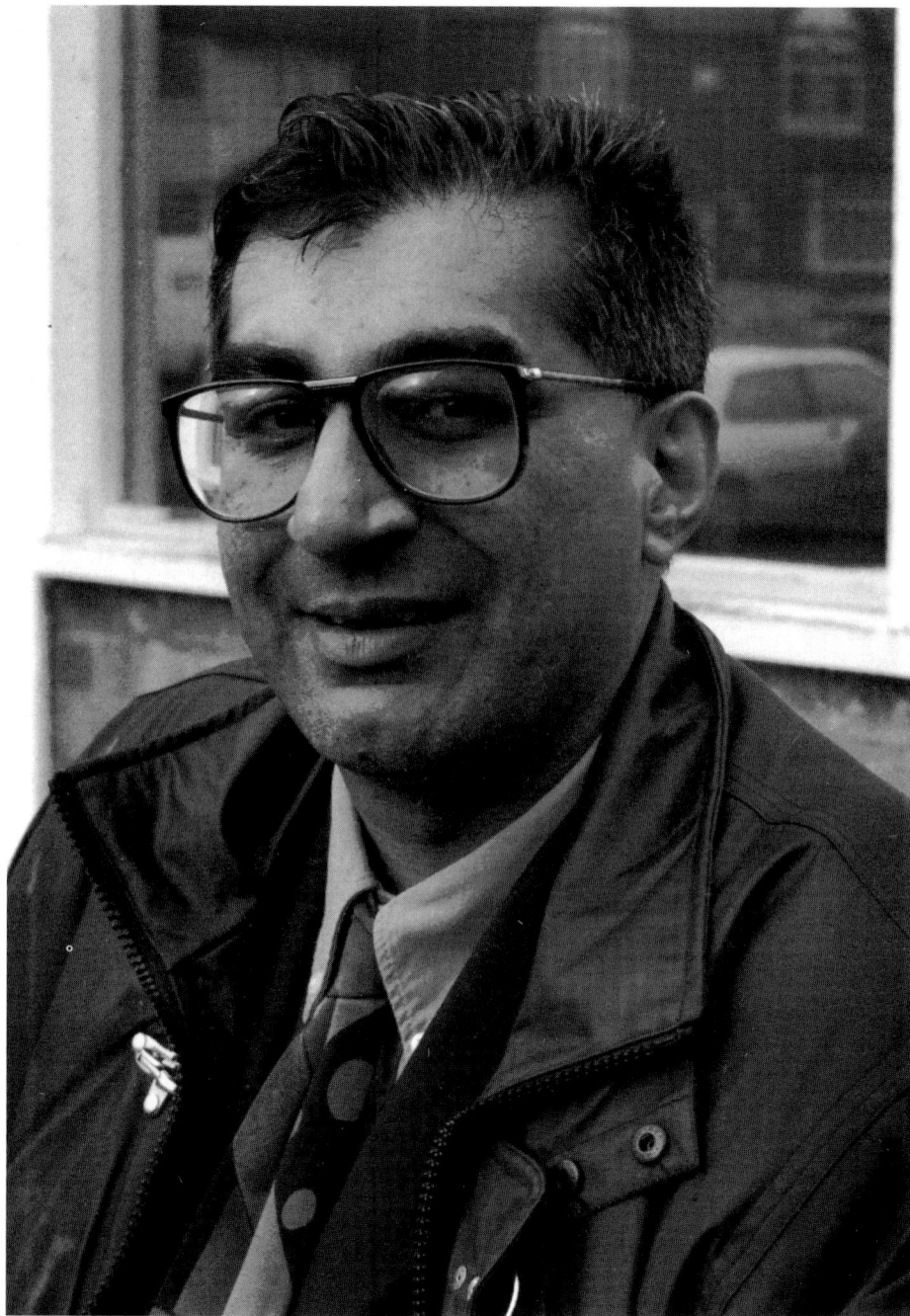

Jagjit Lully was born in Coventry in 1959. He lost both his feet and his right arm to trauma in 1983. He works and is married with two children.

I've been using prosthetics since 1984. I've always come to Oak Tree Lane for my feet and arm. Andy Sharpe has overseen my care. He's brilliant, a very talented person. At the moment he's extremely busy, a piece of elastic band being pulled in different directions. I wouldn't be anywhere without the limb fitting centre. There were people here to help rebuild a life. In trauma, many, many factors come into play. What one individual person needs to rebuild their life is different from another, and the centre has to deal with that variety.

I think I was quite a challenge for the prosthetists here because I have three missing bits and they had to try and make them all work together. I surprised everyone – my rehabilitation was quite straightforward in hindsight. The limbs I had at first were a lot heavier, but the fitting was OK. I know a lot of amputees with all kinds of nightmare problems, but I didn't have many. Within nine months I had a set of limbs and was up and about. I was back working within a year and a half. I accepted the limbs for what they were. It's only later that I thought, 'God, how did I cope with that?' I'm an extremely active person, so I have to be sure that the limbs are functioning all the time. I've got two sets of limbs and I put my trust in the hands of the prosthetists. You have to put your trust in other people when you're disabled. You have to strive to try and do something and you have to take the knocks. Certain people can handle disabilities. A trauma – it's something that's happened, call it 'fate', whatever, it's there.

Upper-arm disabilities are a different level of complexity altogether – I lost mine right up at the shoulder. Even with the latest technology it's extremely difficult to replace a fully functional arm. I was always right handed, but it didn't take long to learn to use my left hand. Obviously there's lots of things that I can't do but the things that I can do are important to keep me functioning. A lot of the adaptations came about naturally, instinctively. I do try and take care of myself, avoid large crowds, watch where I'm walking. You don't take things for granted like an able-bodied person would do. You develop an extra sense to protect yourself.

When I came here I got involved with the running of the centre – I joined the user group to find out about the pressures the prosthetists are under. Words fail me sometimes. I have an insight into the other side of providing this service to us. It's quite an intimate relationship, less formal than many between a hospital and patient. It's not clinical in any way – it was like that even in the 1980s. I've seen the other side of the world, how disability is there, and we're extremely fortunate to have these facilities here. In India and other developing countries there just aren't these services.

You do adapt to a situation; it's a natural instinct, you just have to. Personality comes into it as well, I suppose. People find it hard to cope with anything that's unusual, in all cultures. There've been a lot of hurdles. I was a young man when my accident happened, and it was put to me that you have to think of yourself as being reborn. I've got friends who are quadraplegics, tetraplegics, whatever, it doesn't stop them doing the things that everyone else does. They're a bit philosophical, I suppose, but they don't dwell on it. It's not a nine-to-five preoccupation with what's happened. If that happens it becomes an illness – depression – and they need treatment for it. People do rebuild their lives.

The best way to summarise my attitude is that I've got a humanitarian approach towards people. It's developed over the years, partly through my career, my personality, my parents, what I've seen of the way the world is. I know people from all walks of life, from professionals to the down-trodden, so in that respect I take a balanced view of things. I can see things from different perspectives, different cultural points of view, able-bodied and disabled. I can identify with people who've gone through trauma. I can do that.

People's attitude towards disability depends on many things. Firstly, your own personality and perceptions, life experiences and values. Secondly, it's how you, the disabled person, relate to others. If you play on your disabilities it works against you. Able-bodied people can see that there's things you have problems with, but if you make an issue out of it, that makes them feel guilty. People find it hard to cope with anything that's unusual or not within their own value system. Maturity matters, too. Then there are the blatantly ignorant, who are probably ignorant about lots of things. That's their disability in my opinion.

I've probably achieved more since I became disabled than I did before. There's a 'proving' thing that happens. We live in the 21st century, but the mind-set towards disability goes back centuries. Disabled people in certain cultures are regarded as evil, as having committed sins in the past. Disabled people in western cultures were shunned, locked away, institutionalised. The fear of the bogeyman is present in all walks of life, all cultures. But on the other side there's compassion, the advent of reason. With the advance of technology and modern living the barriers are breaking down. But there's nothing to stop you one day being able-bodied and the next day disabled; the dividing line is very, very fine. Nothing's straightforward, especially in the confused world we live in.

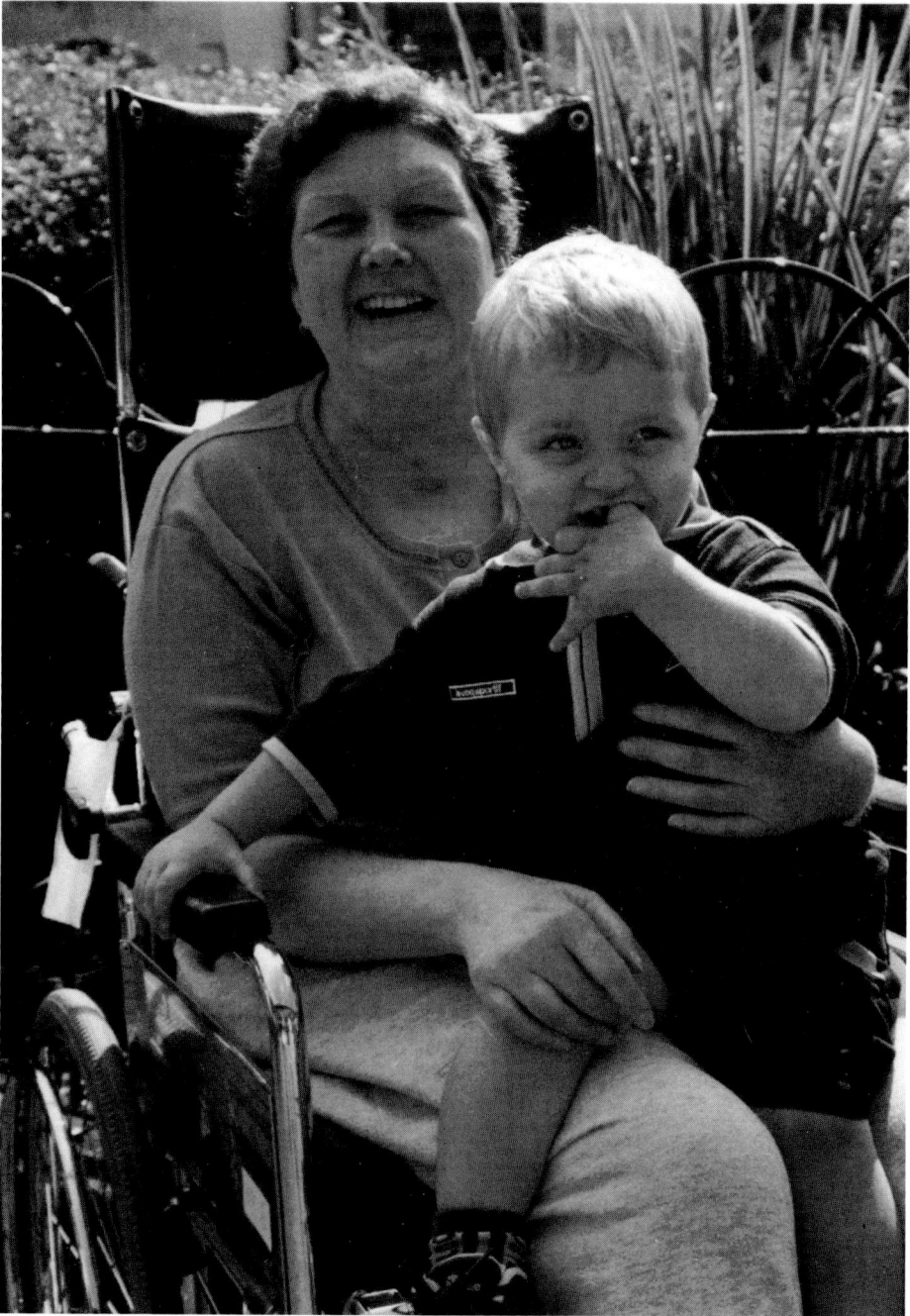

Kathryn Fenn was diagnosed with Guillain-Barré syndrome (GBS) in September 2001. She has three daughters, Alison (23) Laura (21) and Emily (14), and has been in rehab on Ward 3 for four months.

Kathryn: It started off tingling in my gums. I lost my sense of taste – everything tasted like lard. My eyes went and I couldn't stand straight – I was swaying down the street like I'd had a skinful. They sent me to a neurologist and Guillain-Barré syndrome, a virus which sweeps the body, was diagnosed. We didn't know anything about GBS and the girls felt as if they were going in blindfolded. At first I was heavily sedated and can't remember anything, only the bad dreams. Apparently I insulted practically everyone who came to see me.

My daughter Laura is looking after Emily while I'm in rehab and doing really well. She looks after the house and Emily and holds down a full-time job. I keep asking her about the bills and stuff but it's always already sorted. I do worry about them, though. When I was on the ventilator I dreamed I was walking down a road and there were all these dolls face down on the tarmac. If I picked one up, it was one of my three – I shall never forget that.

I settled into Moseley on the first day; everybody was very friendly and helpful. A lady from the GB society came to see me and told me this place was wonderful, magical. Things are going really well but I'm worried about my housing situation – I want the house to be ready for me rather than sitting in here waiting for it. I've got no feeling in the bottom of my legs yet but I'm still hoping to walk out of here. Rehab is exhausting, though. I was so knackered after an OT session on washing and dressing, I slept for the rest of the day. Such a normal thing, but it nearly killed me. But I was so proud of myself that I could wash my hair. Now I set targets from day to day; it's too disappointing if you have long-term targets and don't reach them.

Alison: I had nursed someone with GB so knew that it was possible for Mom to improve. When we knew she was coming to Moseley the staff showed us round, which really put our minds at ease – we looked at all the equipment and the pool. At first I was worried that Mom had MS because I'd seen people with that condition. Here, she's always improving, doing this, doing that. The scariest thing was we were told Mom might come home on a ventilator. Until these things happen to you, you can't say what you'd do or how you'd react. You feel so helpless. I can't imagine my legs not working. As soon as she came off the ventilator, was breathing for herself, I felt better. One day she had six hours off the machine but the next day she was off for 24. You look for tiny improvements at times like that – stupid things, that the machines haven't bleeped so much that night – you hold on to those. We didn't realise exactly what rehab involved, how much Mom would have to re-learn, like brushing her teeth and hair. Mom's got lots to look up to in other patients, like Larry, but then she'll go and see Chris to give him encouragement. They involve the family here, it's really nice: there were no problems with us coming in to organise Emily's party.

Laura: I crashed the car a few days after Mom went into hospital and was desperate to tell her, get it off my chest, but I couldn't for ages because she was so ill. My worst time was when she was in the QE. She used to tell me to get out, that she didn't want to see me. I knew it was the drugs, but I had to explain things to Emily who was crying. I told Emily that Mom was confused, that she didn't mean it. The best is still to come: the hydro pool, the standing and walking frames. At Moseley they let you help a lot more – stuff we might have to do when Mom comes home, which is good. Something like this makes you look at things in perspective – you appreciate things and realise how lucky you are to have the choices we do. I think things will be better than before when she comes home because we won't take things for granted. I used to be so sensitive and would get upset about small things. Now, I don't get so bothered about little things.

Emily: I miss Mom lots. I was counting the days until she came home but I gave up because there were too many; sometimes I feel like an abandoned child. But it's beautiful here. We went out to a pizza place for my birthday tea, I didn't know Mom was going to be there and it was brilliant. If I won the lottery I'd give it to places that do things like this. We've collected money for the GB society. I've had enough of hospitals forever, though. I know that Mom's improving and working towards coming home.

Kathryn: I know there's no pills and potions for GB – you've got to do it yourself. I was concerned that it was hereditary, but there's no more chance of the girls getting it than anyone else. It makes you realise that money's not important. No matter how much money you'd have thrown at me in the QE it wouldn't have made any difference. You've got to have the determination to keep going.

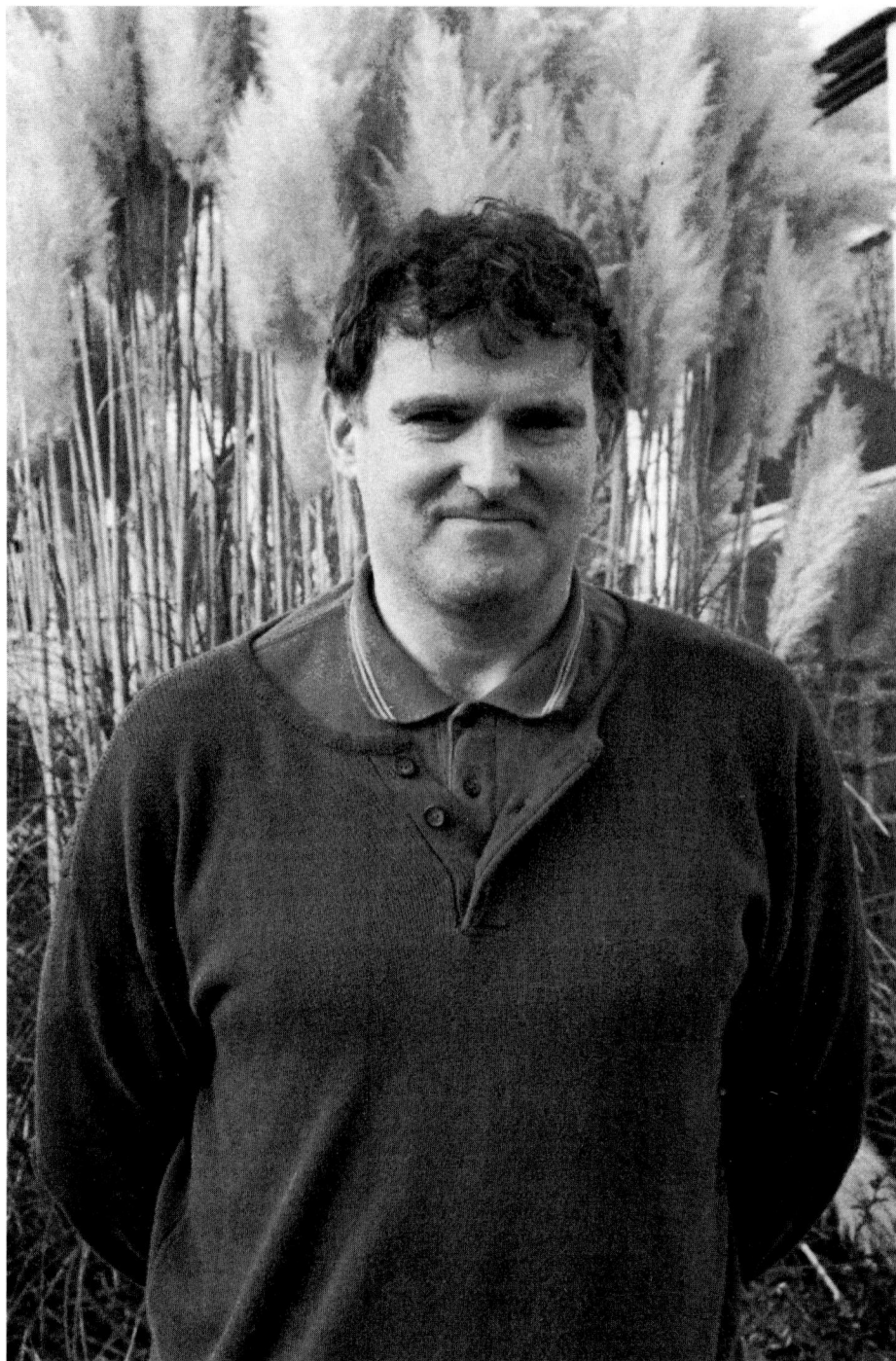

Steve Wilkes was born in West Bromwich in 1961. He lost his right leg above the knee when a car knocked him off his motorbike in 1999. He works as a database manager.

I'd love to say that I came off my bike at 150 miles an hour, but actually I was turning right at a junction and a young kid who'd just passed his test was going too fast to go round the corner. Drove straight into me. All I remember is sitting on my bike, next thing I knew I heard a screeching of brakes and then I remember landing on grass, I remember the smell of the wet grass. I came to some sort of consciousness when the ambulance crew were there and I remember this massive pain, I could feel it coming up from my leg and braced myself ready, because I knew it was coming. I passed out. They kept me sedated for two weeks while they were trying to save my leg. When I woke up it was gone, just like in films. You tell yourself how lucky you are, but on the other hand you think, 'If only I'd been even 10 seconds later or 10 seconds earlier.'

I have a very vivid memory of being told about my leg by a doctor – I think I was told anyway, it's hard to work it out when you're on morphine. I pictured him in a red stripy butcher's apron and he said, 'We had to take your leg off, has nobody told you?' and I said, 'No.' Because I was so spaced out I just said, 'Oh.' That was possibly the worst bit, losing track like that. They'd kept me sedated because they were doing so much work on the leg. But eventually it got infected and that was that. I remember not being able to speak; I couldn't even lift my finger, I was so weak. You're just not in control of your own destiny – it's a horrible feeling.

I've had another complication, I think it's genetic, of excess bone being produced where they tried to pin my hip. I can't move my hip very well and I've also got bony deposits in my stump, which initially was very uncomfortable.

Before the accident I used to run five miles a night. I had a six-pack. The only six-pack I've got now is in the fridge! If you think about it hard, you have to accept that you've lost part of your life. It's hard to adjust, but you have to, otherwise you'd end up having a nervous breakdown. Or become twisted. But human beings can cope, if you don't you're lost. I've started scuba diving again, and I've taken up photography as a replacement for doing bikes, because I used to do a lot of mechanics, rebuild bikes and so on. Photography is technical but it's also artistic as well. I feel like I've got more in touch with an artistic side since my accident; I used to be very mechanical, now I find that I appreciate nature more. Maybe that's a benefit . . .

I wear my leg all day at work. I used to take it off at night and weekends, but now I tend to wear it. Really, I don't like taking it off. People stare at you anyway, I find that difficult to cope with. Taxi drivers seem to think they've got full licence to your life history. I went out with a zimmer frame without my leg, because I didn't have one then, and this little kid just stood there and laughed. I'd have chased after him if I could, whacked him over the head.

They're very good here at Oak Tree Lane, they take a holistic approach. They made sure I went to see the counsellor and so on. Starting a new relationship is the most difficult thing, because I feel so ugly. No one's ever said that to me, but that's how I feel. I don't think there's an answer. You *are* different in society, there's no two ways about it. In the long term I worry about how I'm going to be when I get older. You do see people struggling. It worries me that I'll have to fight for mobility benefits and so on. You shouldn't have to fight for them. That has got me cross.

I just want to strike a balance between being able-bodied but needing a bit of assistance. I've always been somebody who wants to fit in. When you ride a bike you hear about people being killed, losing limbs. But you never think it's going to happen to you. To us, it has happened. I think I'm a bit more sympathetic to people's feelings now, and obviously I understand disability in a totally different way. I understand about exclusion from society, how that happens to people; mental illness – how people get depressed. You understand and can empathise with a much larger range of issues, well I certainly can. So I think from that point of view it has changed me. I was a very insensitive person, now I try and be a bit more sensitive.

You hear people moaning, saying, 'My back hurts, my leg hurts,' and all the rest of it, and you think, 'bloody hell.' People are off work for a couple of months because they've had a broken arm; it does make you more cynical. Overall I think it's made me a slightly better person – but who knows, like with anything in life you change. You might get very frustrated because you've missed out on an opportunity. Best not to do that.

Because I was driven in to and it wasn't my fault there is a feeling that it could happen again. I bought a 4x4 – my black tank – and that's the only vehicle I'll get into. It does stay with you. Your brain says, 'Danger, danger.' I think you've got to be quite a brave person to get back in a vehicle when something like this has happened to you. But if you don't drive you don't have a life.

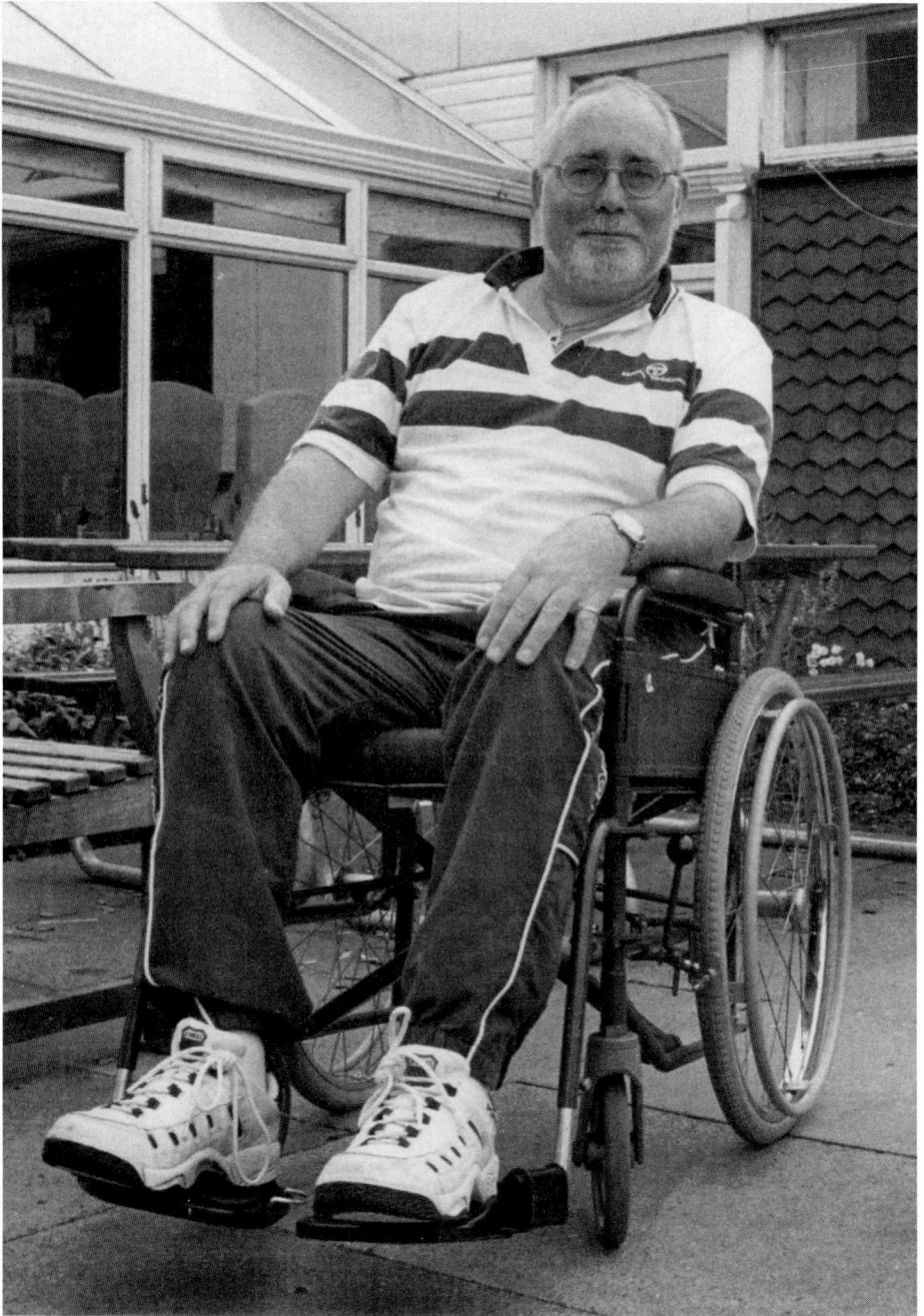

Larry Titmus worked as a sales rep in the packaging industry. He was a keen tennis player, and secretary of Moseley Tennis Club. In March 2002 he was rushed into the QE and subsequently diagnosed with Transverse Myelitis, an inflammation of the fluid in the spinal cord. This interview took place before Larry was walking again – he left ward 3 in September 2002 and now walks without sticks, plays doubles tennis (with a 'fast' partner...), drives and has a new job back in the industry he knows best.

'It's like winning the Olympics, and I couldn't have done it without you, the team.'

Transverse Myelitus is a virus that lies dormant in your body. It's airborne and you can catch it anywhere. It can be in your body for up to 12 months. All of a sudden your immune system will react to it, and from that point the onset is fairly quick.

I first felt it on 7th January, and on 10th March I went down like a sack of ninepins. I didn't feel ill – there wasn't a thing wrong with me above the waist. It was just a numbness, pins and needles like I have now, but my brain couldn't make my legs work. The fear was worse than anything. I haven't walked since then.

The frustration isn't to do with the medical condition – I accept that these things happen – but the unknown quantity of whether I'll walk again. None of the medical staff can give me answers, but no one is working harder than me to get back on my feet, in some form. At this stage I'd be extremely grateful to be on a Zimmer. But ultimately I want nothing less than 100%.

They knew after four days at the QE that I was responding to the drugs because my big toes moved, so they were optimistic that I'd get some mobility back, but no one could say how much. Dr Soyral interviewed me before I came to Moseley to see if I was a suitable candidate for rehab, and he looked me straight in the face and said, 'You know it's likely you'll never play tennis again.' It upset me, but I respect him for it. He said, 'If you hold that in your mind and get used to it, it'll be far better than being told at the last minute, "You aren't going to get any better than this."' I was extremely upset at the time and spent most of the night in tears, but he told me the truth from day one, so I could never be under any illusions. All I can do is give 150%. Since I arrived at Moseley I've gained the greatest respect for everyone here; I didn't think places like this existed. You couldn't pay for this care.

I had another blow on 15th May, in that I lost my job. I asked my wife to read me the letter over the phone, and I was devastated. I'd been taken on to bring in a quarter of a million pounds extra business, and I'd only been with the company for a month when all this happened. I'd settled in well, and then collapsed just outside the office.

The support I've had from this rehab unit is 100%. I cannot fault this place in any form and will sing its praises forever. I've had very low times and the staff have always been supportive. You cross each bridge as you come to it. I'm a salesman and you accept the knockbacks, except this time it's my body and my mind and my future. I may have to retrain and have got one or two irons in the fire. I'm keeping a weekly plan to keep me active in this unit. I've got to be self-motivated.

I have to self-catheterise. People have said, 'You've taken to it like duck to water.' Well – excuse the expression – but who wants to shove a tube up there! In the QE I said, 'You must be joking, I'm not doing that,' and the nurse said, 'You've got two choices: you either do it or you don't. If you don't, you'll have a bag on your leg.' Now I practically do it in my sleep, I don't even think about it. Some people are frightened of things like that. But you have to adapt, take on tasks you never thought you'd have to. In six months' time I'll be thinking, 'I did *that* . . .'

To me, rehabilitation is getting somebody back to the life that they led before. That's it in one sentence, the whole essence of this place. You could write it on the walls. Domestically, socially, emotionally, workwise. Everything is covered in this unit, to get you back into a normal life. For me, it's mainly physio, because if I can walk down this corridor I can walk out of that front door and my life's back. If I can drive a car and see customers, that's acceptable. But then I'll push to be able to run and do social things again – tennis is the ultimate; walks, scuba diving.

There are people who can't go home at weekends, unlike me, and they want the best care they can have and quite rightly so. The other patients on the ward have all been incredibly supportive in all the progress I've made. I really want to thank each and every one of them for that support and encouragement.

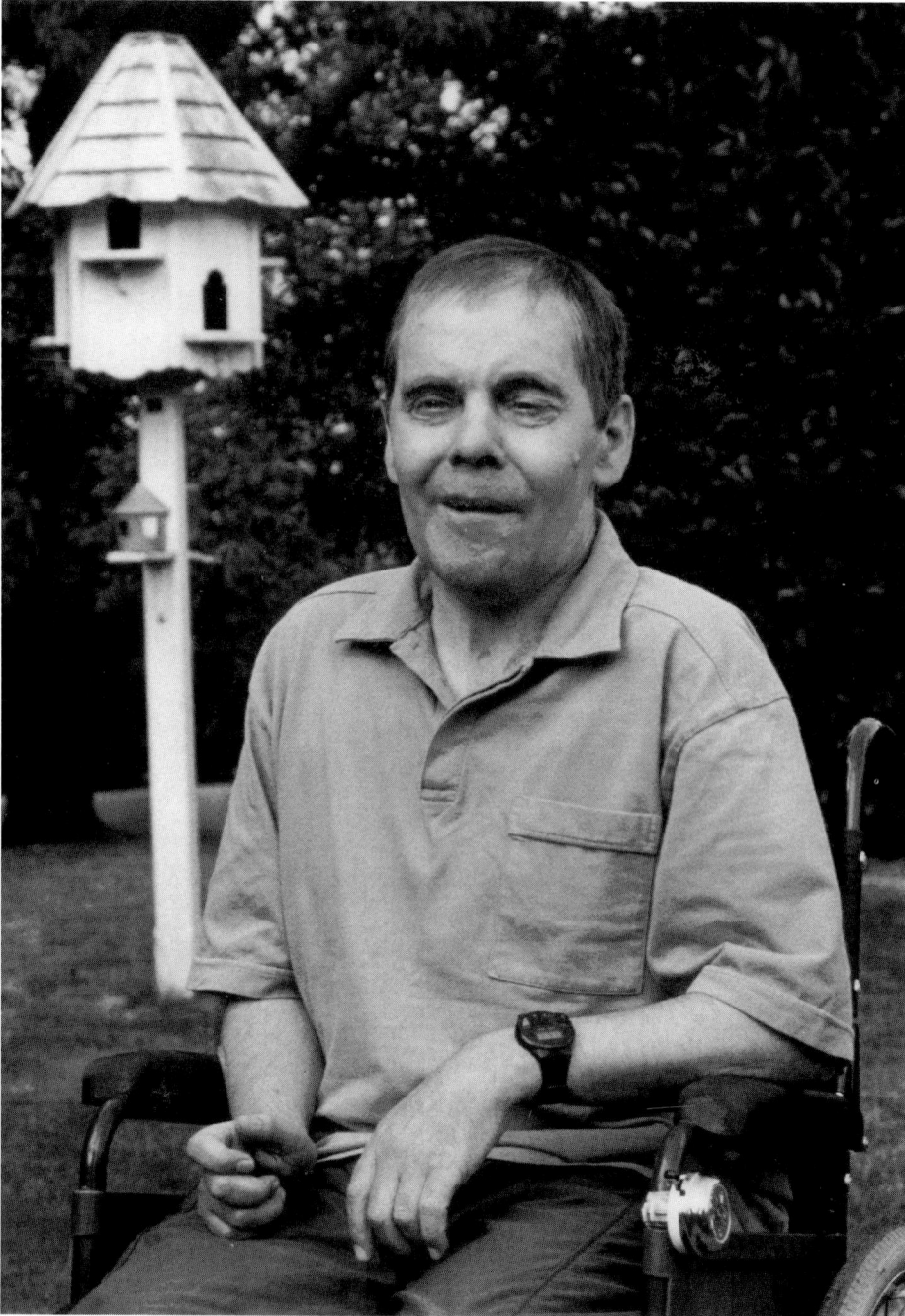

On Tuesday 8th June 1999, Roger Naylor, a keen cyclist, was taking part in a time trial on the A5 in Cannock when he was knocked off his bike by a Frenchman in a Mercedes van delivering quails eggs to Weston Park. Roger suffered very serious head injuries and was taken by air ambulance to Selly Oak Hospital. He was a patient in Hillcrest for over a year and now lives in Leamington Spa.

I don't remember anything about the accident although apparently I was taken to Selly Oak by helicopter – the helicopter pilot came in to visit me later on. I was in a coma in intensive care for approximately two weeks and when I woke up I could only move one finger. I was shocked, but there was hope because something was moving. But I didn't know what to do, how I would manage, what I would do with my life.

I was moved to a trauma ward and gradually came out of my coma. Movement slowly returned to my limbs; I could squeeze my left hand first, but my face was still quite numb. I communicated by pointing to a sheet of letters and spelling out words. But my mind worked faster than my fingers could spell which was very frustrating. Even so, the people who I was 'talking' to sometimes found it hard to keep up.

When I came into Hillcrest I was on a flat bed and people would wheel me about, but the physios were good, they made me move more and got me going. In rehab the physios have to push you – they know what it takes.

At first I couldn't speak properly. I thought I was saying something but

I knew other people couldn't understand me. I thought, 'Bloody hell.' I knew what I wanted to say but the words came out wrong. It was very frightening and I thought, 'What can I do?' I had a typed card to give to new people that I met. It said: *'Please remember I am not deaf or stupid, so put yourself in my place. I have trouble with talking, seeing clearly, balance, swallowing, fatigue. All this is the result of a cycling road accident in June 99. Thank you.'* I used to inadvertently bite my tongue and cheek, but that's better now. Speech and language therapy helped and I worked at it myself. Ironically the hardest word for me to say is speech therapist! But I try really hard. I started to use a wheelchair when I was in Hillcrest; I tried to race in the chair, tired myself out, as if I was in a cycle race . . .

At first I didn't realise my life had changed – I thought I'd get better and go home. It took me a long time to realise things would be different and only now do I recognise that everything has changed forever. Everyone has to adapt in their own way – you have to realise that you're the same person as before but also that you're not. There's a contradiction in your life and you have to live with that.

My family have helped me, my daughters Rachel and Sarah and my wife; my sisters and my brother. They must have found it hard at first, but they've been great. I have a lot of problems which are 'small' in themselves, but all together they add up. It wouldn't be so bad if there were only one problem.

My coping strategies have definitely been other people; other patients because everyone has their moments of sadness. In hospital patients need to talk to each other, to say, 'how are you?' People would say

'OK' when I asked but I knew they weren't, so I'd touch them, reassure them. I made good friends in Hillcrest and have photos of them all.

Now I have small goals as well as big ones. A friend has made me a three-wheel bike that I'm learning to pedal. There are people who've had similar injuries to me who can do it, so I'm going to keep trying. I hope to be able to ride a bike again but it'll be different now, I know that. I need to keep doing physio – the thought of getting on my bike again keeps me going. I want to go up the hills. I'd like to go to Cuba – I like the music – or Jamaica. I also want to be more independent. I can put the music I like and the TV on for myself now, make those choices. I use the computer for email and newsgroups. There's Audaxuk, which is a long-distance cycling newsgroup, and TBIchat for people who've had traumatic brain injuries – it does help to talk to people with the same problems. And email is good for keeping in touch with my family.

I'm eagerly looking forward to the days when I can speak, eat and drink with no problems. As well as ride my bike!

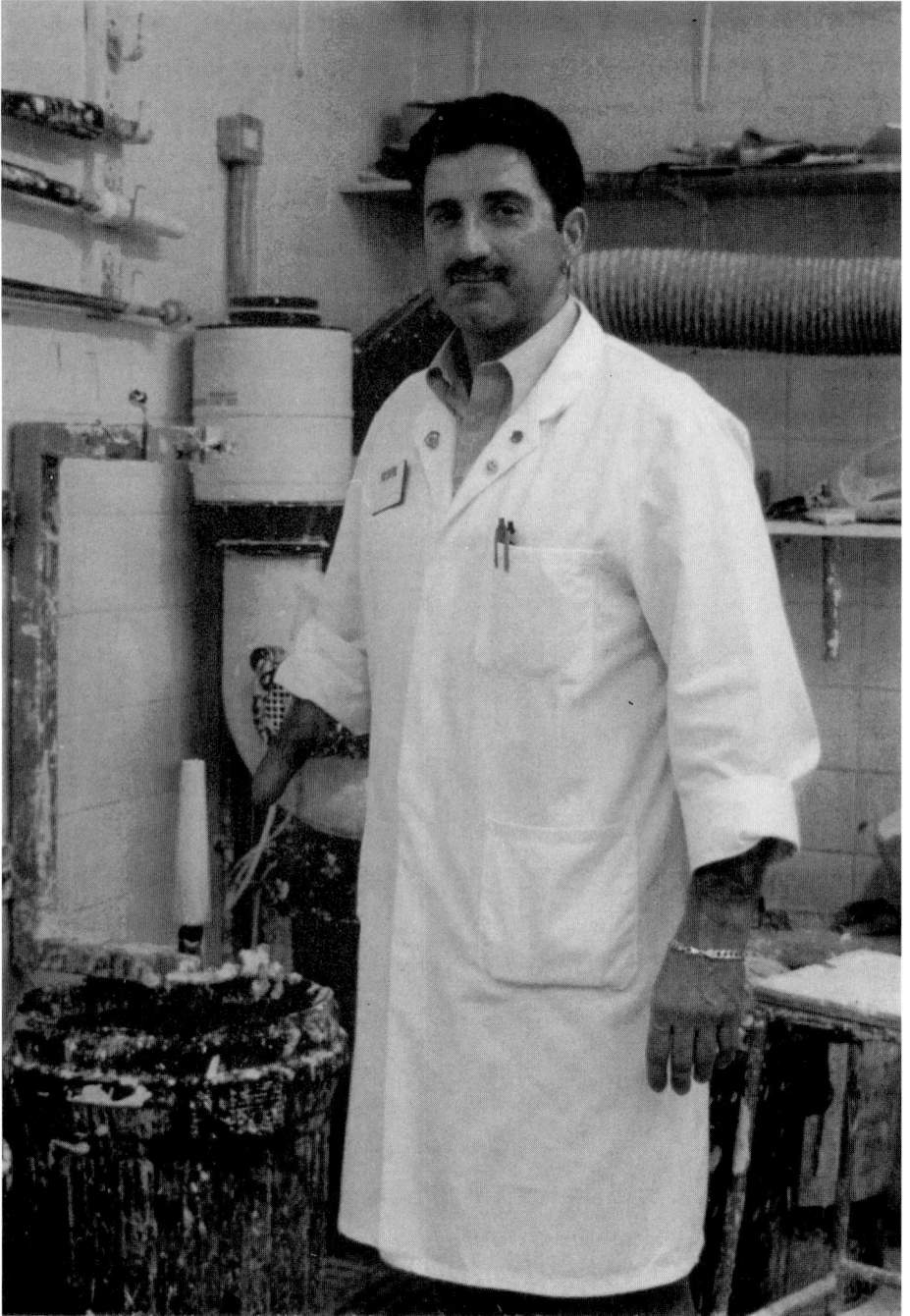

Jim Rainford was born in 1959 in Germany where his father was serving in the Forces. His right hand was missing from birth. He works at Oak Tree Lane Centre as a general clinical assistant and is married with two daughters.

I've been working in the limb trade for 22 years. When I left school I went down the Job Centre and saw an advert for an orderly here. I didn't think I'd get it because of my missing hand. But I got interviewed and had to do a basic test. Part of the job was to work in the basement loading up wheelchairs and I was asked if I'd be able to lift a wheelchair up. I stood up and lifted a chair up with my stump, one-handed. The manager was impressed and realised that my disability wasn't a problem to me. I think that helped me get the job. I've been here ever since. I love the job and I love the people. Being disabled myself, I know what it's like for the patients, I'm in the same boat as them. I was registered as a patient when I got the job here, so I'm both a patient and a member of staff.

I did have an artificial hand when I was a child. I found it handy at times, but very difficult to use at others. My mom encouraged me to try and use it but she didn't make me wear it if I didn't want to. I had old-fashioned arms with a hook on the end, you could pull the hook out, then put in another gadget with a brush or whatever attached. I do everything with my left hand, but can still do a lot with my right arm: push, pull, hit. I'm lucky, my arm's not sensitive, it's very strong and very hard. I adapted quite well as a child. I did find things difficult – tying my shoelaces, putting my tie on. It's hard when you're learning.

I'm a general clinical assistant, so I do anything that the manager or foreman asks me to. I deal with parcels coming into the centre, pack up and send out limbs to patients, keep the workshops and centre as tidy as I can. I also deal with patients and do deliveries. I don't wear an artificial arm at work because I can manage better without it. I do wear my arm occasionally outside work, when I'm wearing a suit, for weddings and special occasions.

Over the years I've got to know lots of the patients here. I've heard some incredible stories – there's a gentleman who's been coming here for years, both his legs were burnt off in a fire. The bedroom ceiling caved in and his legs were trapped dangling into the living room where the fire was. They didn't think he'd ever walk again but he has two artificial limbs and walks very well. That's just one of many stories I could tell.

I had the mickey taken out of me at school, had it all when I was younger: stumpy, one-armed bandit. It's not very nice but you get over that. If I go swimming the children stare, you have to understand that. It's worse with adults because they should know better. There are certain people out there who think you're weird, who look down at you because you've got a disability. Some people are like that. Most of my friends and family look at me when I *am* wearing my artificial arm. They say, 'What are you wearing that for?'

Children always ask, 'How did you lose your arm, mate?' Nine times out of ten I just tell them I was born like this and they say, 'Why?' and I say, 'It's just one of those things, it happens.' And it still does. I don't think there'll ever be a cure for that.

Most of the people here manage very well with their lives. A lot of it is mental, getting to an understanding that you've got to carry on your life without your limbs. Sometimes it's very hard though. There are people who have problems – nothing runs smoothly in this world and no two people are the same, no two amputations are the same, no two limbs are the same.

I enjoy the job because I work with a lot of nice people. We come here to do a job, to supply and look after artificial limbs for people who need them, so that's satisfying in itself. Amputees will always need limbs until they die. I might stop working here one day but I'll still be a patient here, still have to come back for repairs or whatever. It's a lifetime relationship.

I could have had a myoelectric arm, but the motor's a couple of inches long and then you've got the hand on the end of it. My artificial arm would be longer than my other arm. Until they can make a battery that can fit into the actual hand I'll adapt to how things are. The hook was the most useful tool I ever had but it wasn't very pretty. People still wear them, if they work in factories and need to do a special job. You can get arms with a rest on for playing snooker now! I've got a socket the shape of my stump on the handlebar of my mountain bike, it rotates. I put my stump in and I can steer without the stump slipping off.

My number one hobby is football. I've played football since I was 15 and I'm a big Manchester United supporter. I follow them everywhere. All the home games: I've got a season ticket and go to Old Trafford every couple of weeks. I went to Barcelona for the European Cup Final. I was there. I used to play at the weekends, for Colinthians in the Birmingham AFA league. At school I played basketball and – wait for this – cricket. I held the bat and used my stump at the top end to lean it against, and was able to control it there. I wasn't too bad a batter. I didn't let my disability get in my way, and the teachers helped me. I played centre-forward, and I've played in goal four times for various teams and only lost once. Once I was in goal and 20 minutes into the game one of their strikers turned round and said to our left-back, 'Are you taking the mickey out of us? Your guy's only got one hand!' I think he swore actually.

Pat Tovey was born in Kidderminster in 1959, a thalidomide baby. She had multiple operations as a child and her right leg was eventually amputated in 1980. She is married with two daughters, Natasha and Michaela, and is currently studying for five A Levels.

Basically I was born thalidomide, my right leg hadn't developed, the foot was a club foot and facing the wrong way – I had four operations before I was six to get it round. I used to wear surgical boots and calipers. My father died when I was two, and I had a mother who didn't care about me. School was very grim. The kids picked on me, they used to sing, 'Pat's got the lurgy.' The lads were very, very cruel, worse than the girls, but as we got older the girls got crueller. I was the outcast, and that was it. I used to steal sweets from the shop just to give to people, so they'd be my friends for a few minutes, that's how bad my life was. I'd love to have a class reunion now and go back and hold my head up high.

When I was 11 my mum took me to another hospital and they said, 'The best thing for this child would be to remove the leg,' but she wouldn't have it. When I was 15 I had my leg lengthened four inches. They cut the bone and turned this knob every day to pull it apart. But the new bone wouldn't knit. I spent six years on crutches.

I met my first husband, Chris, when I was 15. He was a bad 'un, but I had Natasha by that marriage, a week before my 21st birthday. I used to do everything on crutches: push the pram, get my shopping, do the housework, peg the washing out, even go out dancing. I used to hop onto the dance floor, deposit my crutches against the wall, and dance all night long on one leg. My left leg's amazing. Amazing. It's never let me down. After I had Natasha I decided to have the leg removed – the hospital said, 'I think that would be a good thing.' I should have had my leg taken off when I was younger – I'd have fitted in better at school and I certainly wouldn't have missed out on so much education. I do say one thing for my mother, though, she did fight for me to go to a normal school. In all, I had 18 operations. When I used to go to the Woodlands they'd say, 'We've got your bed warm for you, Pat.' I was happier in hospital than anywhere else, it was my second home. I know it sounds silly, but when I was in hospital there were people there who cared about me. The staff cared.

On 12th December 1980, I had my leg removed. It was the best day of my life. I wasn't joyful for the leg being gone, it's when I look back now that I know. When I went down to theatre they didn't know if they were going to remove it above or below the knee, so when I came round and I'd still got my knee, I was delighted. It was the beginning of my life.

After the Woodlands I came to Selly Oak and was introduced to Andrew Perry. I was to become one of his patients – he still hasn't got rid of me! Andrew made me a leg. It wasn't a very nice leg: a brown leather socket with laces at the back and two metal rods. But I still felt great because I'd got proper shoes on both feet – they weren't overly nice shoes, but shoes.

I decided to alter, then. I had my hair highlighted and permed, my ears pierced, started to wear make-up. I lost all my weight. In the meantime, Andrew made me this lovely leg. I could wear four-inch heels. I started off at about two inches, then I'd go up to three, he'd be wiping his head, going, 'Oh God.' I used to come into the centre like a pop star, with my sunglasses and my long hair, skirts up to my thighs and over-the-knee boots like *Pretty Woman*. I did cause a lot of grief for Andrew, I think. But I'd missed out on all those years. I was working in sales. I was a croupier at Dudley Casino. I had my own house, I was doing very well. Basically I think I was proving to myself that I was desirable, that my disability wouldn't be a problem. I used to go out all the time, clubbing. There was one bloke who'd been chasing me round the nightclub, and it got to the stage where he said, 'Do you want to come back to mine?' I said, 'I'm not like other women,' and he said, 'You're not a man, are you!' It didn't put him off. I've always said, 'I've got all my working bits, my womanly bits.'

My life began the day my leg came off. All the rest of it has been like watching something on the television. The calipers went. I looked in the mirror and I saw two legs, two shoes, and I thought, 'I'm not ugly now.' I've always felt as if my life deserved more.

Dancing is my passion. I'm always the first one on the dance floor. I know I'm a good dancer. When I'm on the dance floor I feel so alive. I only have to hear that beat, and off I go. Once I'd had an operation on my leg and I went to the nightclub, I'd only been out of hospital for 10 days. I said to my friends, 'Whatever you do, don't let me dance,' but as soon as I heard the beat I was gone. It hurt, but it was worth it. I can spin round and round and round on one leg. Andrew says, 'No dancing,' but he knows that I'm my own worst enemy.

Having my leg off has improved my life. When I see people I try to give them inspiration, and I think I do. Everybody has just got to be determined to live. I'm living proof that you can have a life from nothing. I've remarried, I'm settled and very happy. I've still got to have a goal and that's why I've gone to college. Now I have a brilliant life; people would like to swap their life for mine.

Eric Minchin was born in Stepney in 1927, and was evacuated to Worcester in 1940. He had an above-knee amputation aged eight and walked, cycled and even ran on his peg-leg, not bothering with a foot until he started courting. He has two children and two grandchildren.

I can't remember much about my life before the amputation. I remember having a double-barrelled pop gun for Christmas, that's about it. All I had was a kick at school, which caused osteomyelitis. I don't think there was even a mark on my leg. I cried a bit; it was very painful. I went into hospital and stayed there until they took it off, about 18 months later. The osteomyelitis was in the shin, and as it progressed up the body they said it's either that or amputate. Sir Hamilton Bailey from Harley Street took it off – we had to go private, cost my dad a small fortune. In those days it was five guineas to stand by the bed, there was no NHS. By all accounts I never cried until the very last time that I went into the operating theatre. Whether I knew something I don't know.

I've never had any trouble whatsoever since; no pain, nothing. The first leg I had was a wooden peg-leg with a carved socket. Round at the bottom, no foot on it or anything, about two inches in diameter. My father took me up to Oxford Street. He turned round and I'd disappeared but there was a great big crowd. My leg had gone down the grating. They were trying to pull me out but they didn't realise it wasn't hurting me. The peg-leg was really jammed 'cos I'd gone down with a wallop.

I could run, walk, climb with my peg-leg. What with hospital, convalescence and then the war I didn't get much schooling. The family got bombed out of Stepney about 1940, just before the doodlebug started. My father had 24 hours leave and came up to the dugout –

we lived there because there was a raid every night – and took us to Paddington Station. It seemed to take about five days just to get to Oxford. We'd never been on a train. There was Granny, with her hat and gas mask on. There was Mother – she was pregnant. There was my younger brother; me with my peg-leg and a dog on a bit of string. It was like a Giles cartoon.

I woke up in the morning and there was this terrible noise and I thought, 'What the blazes is that?' I looked out of the window and there were these great big animals – cows, but I'd never seen one before. There were about 80 of these things.

To me, I wasn't disabled – I'd got a wooden leg and that was the end of it. But when my father came home on leave he did his nut that I was working in a quarry with one leg. I was taken on as an apprentice bookbinder by Ebeneezer Bayliss in Worcester. It was a wonderful job because it wasn't like work. I used to do the big leather-bound account books: gold-edged, marble-edged, gold leaf and gold tooling. That's when I first started cycling, because I had to, to get to work: 12 miles there and 12 miles back.

After the war I cycled all over Europe, staying in youth hostels. The peg-leg hung over the side and I cycled with one leg. No problem. I'd say to my mother, 'I'm just nipping down to London,' and go to my aunt's in Catford. The most I ever did in one hop was 189 miles. My leg was like a piston, up and down all day long. It was wonderful. I'd beat the guys with two legs. We'd cycle to Paris quite easily. I fancied cycling round the world. We cycled to Harwich and then through Belgium, Holland, Denmark and France. We were hoping to work our way round. I had about a tenner.

I lived on a boat for two years – a Fairmile B, the motor torpedo boats. That was a good time. We were on the River Severn. This chap had bought it and wanted to convert it so we could sail. There were three ladies, three men – no hanky-panky – we got on quite well. All the men worked solid on the boat and the women went to work to get the money.

I was very fit then and the strength was in my arms. I could climb anything providing I had something to hang on to. I went mountain climbing in Switzerland. Once the peg-leg was down you could put 10 ton on it. It did use to sink into things, though. I worked on a farm when we first got bombed out of Stepney. I used to walk along and they'd follow me and drop spuds in the holes! The leg I wear now must be 30-odd years old – made in Corporation Street, I used to cycle up there. I only go to Selly Oak for socks and to get it fixed. I've worn an artificial limb for 65 years and have never had any problems except for when it breaks. There's nothing I can't do. I built my extension; if anyone around here wants anything doing with their roof they call me.

I read in the paper that a 12-year-old lad had been run over by a tractor in Droitwich and lost a leg. I thought, 'Ideal opportunity for me to try and impart some of my knowledge.' So I phoned up the hospital and they said they'd have a word with his mother. I went and befriended him, took him fishing, one thing or another. He got on quite well, but the first leg he had was just hanging off him. I keep my belts really tight. Immediately I move the leg moves. I tried it without the shoulder strap but I can't walk fast enough without it. This leg is so positive, it's all metal, there's no give in it at all. The only regret in my life is that I stopped cycling.

Editor's note:
Eric Minchin is pictured on the back cover.